Cancer Pharmacology and Pharmacotherapy Review

Cancer Pharmacology and Pharmacotherapy Review

Study Guide for Oncology Boards and MOC Exams

Francis P. Worden, MD, RPh
Professor
Division of Hematology/Oncology
Department of Internal Medicine
University of Michigan Health System
Ann Arbor, Michigan

Anthony J. Perissinotti, PharmD, BCOP
Clinical Pharmacist Specialist, Inpatient Hematology
Adjunct Clinical Assistant Professor
Department of Pharmacy
University of Michigan Health System
Ann Arbor, Michigan

Bernard L. Marini, PharmD
Clinical Pharmacist Specialist, Inpatient Hematology
Adjunct Clinical Assistant Professor
Department of Pharmacy
University of Michigan Health System
Ann Arbor, Michigan

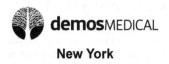

demosMEDICAL

New York

Visit our website at www.demosmedical.com
ISBN: 9781620700761
e-book ISBN: 9781617052521

Acquisitions Editor: David D'Addona
Compositor: Exeter Premedia Services

Medicine is an ever-changing science. Research and clinical experience are continually expanding our knowledge, in particular our understanding of proper treatment and drug therapy. The authors, editors, and publisher have made every effort to ensure that all information in this book is in accordance with the state of knowledge at the time of production of the book. Nevertheless, the authors, editors, and publisher are not responsible for errors or omissions or for any consequences from application of the information in this book and make no warranty, expressed or implied, with respect to the contents of the publication. Every reader should examine carefully the package inserts accompanying each drug and should carefully check whether the dosage schedules mentioned therein or the contraindications stated by the manufacturer differ from the statements made in this book. Such examination is particularly important with drugs that are either rarely used or have been newly released on the market.

Library of Congress Cataloging-in-Publication Data
Names: Worden, Francis P., author. | Perissinotti, Anthony J., author. |
  Marini, Bernard L., author.
Title: Cancer pharmacology and pharmacotherapy review : study guide for
  oncology boards and MOC exams / Francis P. Worden, Anthony J.
  Perissinotti, Bernard L. Marini.
Description: New York : Demos Medical, [2016]
Identifiers: LCCN 2015045238 | ISBN 9781620700761 | ISBN 9781617052521
  (ebook)
Subjects: | MESH: Antineoplastic Agents—pharmacology—Examination Questions.
  | Neoplasms—drug therapy—Examination Questions.
Classification: LCC RS431.A64 | NLM QV 18.2 | DDC 615.7/98076—dc23
LC record available at http://lccn.loc.gov/2015045238

Printed in the United States of America by McNaughton & Gunn.
16 17 18 19 / 5 4 3 2 1

We dedicate this book to our patients for their willingness to participate in clinical trials. Without their fortitude and willingness to participate in clinical trials, new drug discoveries and the advancement of the field of oncologic medicine would not be possible.

Contents

List of Figures

List of Tables

Preface

In preparing for clinics, rounding, or board examinations, understanding the pharmacology of the drugs and agents can be overwhelming. In medical school and residency, it is often difficult to keep up with the mechanisms of action, kinetics, and dosing schedules of so many common medications, let alone those that are used in more rare conditions, including cancer. When residents become hematology and oncology fellows, they are forced to learn a large cohort of medications very quickly, a task that is daunting, given the ever-expanding market of new chemotherapeutic agents.

Additionally, questions on the hematology and oncology board examinations related to pharmacology represent a relatively larger percentage. This is true, given that the facts focusing on the mechanisms and side effects of these drugs do not change. Moreover, we are often asked dose-limiting side effects of medications as well as the requirements for dosage reductions related to kidney and liver failure. The University of Michigan Hematology/Oncology Fellowship Program recently published an oncology board review book, *Oncology Boards Flash Review*, to help solidify the knowledge one needs to have for his or her test. As a companion to this manual, we have written a similar board review book to summarize information that is most pertinent to the pharmacology of chemotherapeutic agents used by practicing hematologists and oncologists. This book contains concise summaries of the various chemotherapeutic drugs by class, pharmacology, pharmacokinetics, and toxicities and includes, to date, all of the U.S. Food and Drug Administration (FDA)-approved oncology agents available to practicing clinicians. It is our hope that fellows and practicing medical hematologists/oncologists preparing for ward rounds, outpatient clinical rotations, or for their certification or recertification examinations will find our book to be a useful tool. Our goal is to help our readers summarize and solidify many important clinical facts and to help them build confidence in their knowledge of oncologic drugs.

The successful completion of this project was made possible by the editorial staff of Demos Medical Publishing, especially David D'Addona, acquisitions editor, and Joseph Stubenrauch, production editor.

Francis P. Worden, MD, RPh
Anthony J. Perissinotti, PharmD, BCOP
Bernard L. Marini, PharmD

Traditional Chemotherapy

Microtubule Inhibitors

TAXANES AND RELATED AGENTS

What are the chemotherapy agents in the taxane class?

- Paclitaxel (Taxol®), nanoparticle albumin-bound (nab) paclitaxel (Abraxane®), docetaxel (Taxotere®), and cabazitaxel (Jevtana®)
- Ixabepilone (Ixempra®) is an epothilone
- Eribulin (Halaven®) is a halichondrin B analogue

What malignancies are each taxane FDA approved for?

FDA-Approved Uses of Taxanes

Agent	FDA Approval
Paclitaxel	Breast cancer, non–small cell lung cancer (NSCLC), ovarian cancer, Kaposi's sarcoma
Nab-paclitaxel	Breast cancer, pancreatic cancer, NSCLC
Docetaxel	Breast cancer, NSCLC, prostate cancer, gastric adenocarcinoma, head and neck cancers
Cabazitaxel	Prostate (post-docetaxel)
Ixabepilone	Metastatic breast cancer
Eribulin	Metastatic breast cancer

Abbreviation: FDA, U.S. Food and Drug Administration.

How do the taxanes work? (See Figure 1.1)

- Summary: More microtubule assembly occurs than disassembly, resulting in abnormal arrays or bundles of microtubules throughout the cell cycle leading to apoptosis (primarily via caspase 9 activation)

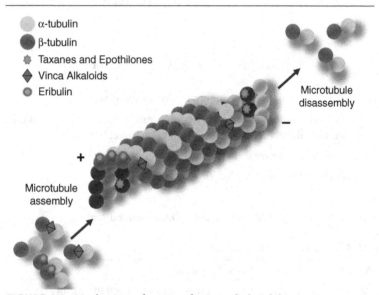

○ α-tubulin
● β-tubulin
✿ Taxanes and Epothilones
◆ Vinca Alkaloids
◉ Eribulin

Microtubule disassembly

+ Microtubule assembly

−

FIGURE 1.1. Mechanism of action of microtubule inhibitors: As a class, microtubule inhibitors interfere with microtubule dynamics and the formation of the mitotic spindle, thus preventing cell cycle progression from the G2→M phase, ultimately leading to apoptosis. Vinca alkaloids prevent microtubule assembly by binding β-tubulin and promoting depolymerization. Eribulin binds to a site near the vinca-binding site, preventing microtubule assembly and causing formation of nonproductive tubulin aggregates. Uniquely, eribulin binds only to the "plus" end of microtubules and does not affect microtubule shortening. Taxanes bind to β-tubulin on the interior surface of microtubules, promoting stabilization of the microtubule and preventing dissociation of tubulin. Epothilones have a similar mechanism of action to taxanes and occupy the same binding site; however, they interact with β-tubulin through a different molecular binding mechanism.

- Microtubules lengthen and shrink via attachment/detachment of α- and β-tubulin dimers. In a normal cell, there is a dynamic equilibrium of polymerization and depolymerization. This is termed *dynamic instability*. Taxanes block dynamic instability by binding to β-tubulin, causing less detachment of α- and β-tubulin dimers and more stability of the microtubules, leading them to be shifted to the assembled state. When more assembly occurs than disassembly, abnormal bundles of microtubules result and cellular function and replication cannot proceed

- Cell cycle specific to the G2/M phase

How do the mechanisms of nab-paclitaxel, cabazitaxel, ixabepilone, and eribulin differ?

- Nab-paclitaxel: preferentially delivers paclitaxel out of serum and into tumor interstitium via interactions with albumin receptors. In addition, serum protein acidic that is rich in cysteine (SPARC) can be overexpressed on tumors, which nab-paclitaxel can bind to, resulting in the tumor cell rapidly internalizing paclitaxel

- Cabazitaxel: poor affinity for the P-glycoprotein (P-gp) efflux pump, therefore active in cell lines that are resistant to paclitaxel/docetaxel and achieves greater central nervous system concentrations

- Ixabepilone: exhibits greater potency binding to paclitaxel binding site via different molecular interactions and is not affected by mutations in β-tubulin that cause resistance to taxanes; maintains activity despite tumors overexpressing P-gp, βIII-tubulin, and microtubule assembly proteins; also enhances caspase-2-induced apoptosis

- Eribulin: inhibits microtubule assembly without affecting disassembly by binding soluble tubulin (causing formation of aggregates) and binding to the growing (+) end of the microtubule

What are common mechanisms of resistance to taxane therapy?

- Alterations in the α- and β-tubulin subunits can decrease the rate of polymerization into microtubules

- Overexpression of the MDR1 gene, which encodes for a membrane P-gp efflux pump

- Overexpression of βIII-tubulin and microtubule assembly proteins
- Interactions of microtubules with other cytoskeletal proteins
- Defects in apoptotic pathways

What are the common dosing ranges for each taxane?

- Paclitaxel: 50 to 200 mg/m^2 intravenous (IV) over 1 to 3 hours or up to 250 mg/m^2 IV over 24 hours every 3 weeks
- Nab-paclitaxel: 100 to 125 mg/m^2 IV over 30 minutes on days 1, 8, and 15 of 21- to 28-day cycle; 260 mg/m^2 IV over 30 minutes every 3 weeks
- Docetaxel: adult: 60 to 100 mg/m^2 IV over 1 hour every 3 weeks; pediatric sarcomas: 75 to 125 mg/m^2; 30 to 40 mg/m^2 IV weekly for 3 weeks every 28 days
- Cabazitaxel: 25 mg/m^2 IV over 1 hour every 3 weeks in combination with prednisone (10 mg orally (PO) once daily continuously)
- Ixabepilone: 40 mg/m^2 IV over 3 hours every 3 weeks; max body surface area (BSA) 2.2 m^2
- Eribulin: 1.4 mg/m^2 IV over 2 to 5 minutes on days 1 and 8 every 21 days

What solvents are the taxanes in and why is this important?

- Paclitaxel: Cremophor® EL (use non–polyvinyl chloride [PVC] tubing, bag, and connectors; 0.2 to 1.2 micron in-line filter required)
- Nab-paclitaxel: delivered in an amorphous, nanoparticle form to overcome insolubility in aqueous solutions (no cremophor or polysorbate 80; no special tubing; in-line filter is not recommended)
- Docetaxel: polysorbate 80 (use non-PVC tubing, bag, and connectors; in-line filter not recommended)
- Cabazitaxel: polysorbate 80 (use non-PVC tubing, bag, and connectors; 0.2 to 1.2 micron in-line filter required)
- Ixabepilone: cremophor (use non-PVC bag, tubing, and connectors; 0.2 to 1.2 micron in-line filter)
- Eribulin: does not contain solvents such as cremophor or polysorbate 80 (non-PVC equipment, in-line filter not required)

– Cremophor leads to immediate hypersensitivities (monitor patient's vital signs every 15 minutes during infusion; reactions usually occur within the first 10 minutes of infusion)

– Polysorbate 80 leads to delayed hypersensitivities such as fluid accumulations

Are the taxanes metabolized/eliminated renally or hepatically?

- All four taxanes are extensively metabolized hepatically
- All four taxanes (except eribulin) do not appear to require dose adjustments for renal dysfunction

Are there drug interactions with any of the taxanes?

Taxanes should be administered prior to platinum derivatives to limit myelosuppression and enhance efficacy

- Paclitaxel: affected by CYP3A4 and CYP2C8 inhibitors/inducers, P-gp inhibitors; sequence doxorubicin/epirubicin prior to paclitaxel as paclitaxel can increase the maximum concentration (Cmax) and decrease clearance of these agents resulting in profound neutropenia and stomatitis; sequence paclitaxel prior to cyclophosphamide to reduce myelosuppression
- Nab-paclitaxel: not well characterized; assumed to be similar to paclitaxel
- Docetaxel: affected by CYP3A4 inhibitors/inducers, radiotherapy (radiation recall and radiosensitization); sequence doxorubicin/epirubicin/vinorelbine/topotecan before docetaxel to reduce profound neutropenia
- Cabazitaxel: affected by CYP3A4 inhibitors/inducers
- Ixabepilone: affected by CYP3A4 inhibitors/inducers
- Eribulin: a CYP3A4 inhibitor and weak inhibitor of P-gp; thus will affect substrates of CYP3A4 and P-gp

What are the class adverse effects of the taxanes?

- Infusion reactions
- Myelosuppression

- Neuropathy
- Alopecia (generally full body)
- Myalgia
- Fatigue

What are the most common adverse effects of each taxane?

- Paclitaxel: myelosuppression (more thrombocytopenia), cardiovascular and hypersensitivity reactions (characterized by hypotension, dyspnea, flushing, and rash), peripheral sensory neuropathy, central nervous system (CNS) effects from dehydrated alcohol, alopecia, skin reactions, bradycardia, and radiation recall

- Nab-paclitaxel: myelosuppression (less thrombocytopenia), peripheral sensory neuropathy (appears more reversible than paclitaxel), alopecia, edema, skin rash, hypersensitivity (rare), and ocular disturbances (blurred vision and photopsia)

- Docetaxel: fluid retention (peripheral edema, generalized edema, pleural effusions, dyspnea at rest, cardiac tamponade, or pronounced abdominal distention due to ascites), myelosuppression (more than paclitaxel), cutaneous reactions, less cardiotoxicity than paclitaxel, peripheral neuropathy, conjunctivitis, lacrimation, stomatitis/mucositis, diarrhea, hepatotoxicity, and myalgias/arthralgias

- Cabazitaxel: myelosuppression, febrile neutropenia, fatigue, urinary tract infections, dehydration, less hypersensitivity reactions, diarrhea, acute renal failure (from diarrhea/dehydration), less peripheral neuropathy, less alopecia, minimal fluid retention, minimal onychodystrophy

- Ixabepilone: peripheral neuropathy, CNS effects (high concentration of dehydrated alcohol), radiation recall, myelosuppression, less hypersensitivity, constipation, stomatitis/mucositis, anorexia, alopecia, and arthralgias/myalgias

- Eribulin: peripheral neuropathy, myelosuppression, febrile neutropenia, QT prolongation, anorexia, arthralgias/myalgias, decreased liver function, and alopecia

What is the difference in the side effect profile between weekly dosing and dosing every 3 weeks of paclitaxel and docetaxel?

Differences in Side Effect Profile Between Weekly Dosing and Dosing Every 3 Weeks of Paclitaxel and Docetaxel

	Weekly	Every 3 Weeks
Paclitaxel	Nail/skin changes	Myelosuppression
	Edema	More alopecia (total body loss)
	Neuropathy (but delayed)	Myalgia
	Generally better tolerated	*Continuous infusion:* more myelosuppression, mucositis, diarrhea, febrile neutropenia, possibly less neuropathy
Docetaxel	Tear duct changes	Myelosuppression
	Nail/skin changes	Mucositis
	Hand-foot syndrome	Myalgia

What are the premedications required?

Premedications Required for Taxanes

Drug	Premedication
Paclitaxel	Dexamethasone 20 mg IV, diphenhydramine 50 mg IV, and famotidine 20 mg IV
Nab-paclitaxel	None required
Docetaxel	1. Dexamethasone (8 mg PO twice daily for 3 days starting 1 day prior to treatment) 2. Prostate cancer: dexamethasone (8 mg PO at 12 hr, 3 hr, and 1 hr prior to the docetaxel infusion) 3. Simplified: 20 mg IV dexamethasone
Cabazitaxel	Dexamethasone 10 mg IV, diphenhydramine 50 mg IV, and famotidine 20 mg IV
Ixabepilone	Diphenhydramine 50 mg IV and famotidine 20 mg IV
Eribulin	None

What is the emetogenicity level of the taxanes?

- All six agents are categorized as low

Are the taxanes vesicants or irritants?

- Paclitaxel: irritant with vesicantlike properties
- Nab-paclitaxel: irritant
- Docetaxel: irritant
- Cabazitaxel: irritant
- Ixabepilone: irritant
- Eribulin: nonvesicant/nonirritant

VINCA ALKALOIDS

What are the chemotherapy agents in the vinca alkaloid class?

- Vincristine (Oncovin®)
- Liposomal vincristine (Marqibo®)
- Vinblastine (Velban®)
- Vinorelbine (Navelbine®)

What malignancies are each vinca alkaloid FDA approved for?

FDA-Approved Uses of Vinca Alkaloids

Agent	FDA Approval
Vincristine	Acute lymphoblastic leukemia (ALL), Hodgkin's (HL) and non-Hodgkin's lymphoma (NHL), Wilms' tumor, neuroblastoma, rhabdomyosarcoma
Liposomal vincristine	ALL
Vinblastine	HL and NHL, testicular cancer, breast cancer, Kaposi's sarcoma, histiocytosis, choriocarcinoma
Vinorelbine	Non–small cell lung cancer

Abbreviation: FDA, U.S. Food and Drug Administration.

How do the vinca alkaloids work? (See Figure 1.1)

- Derived from the Madagascar periwinkle plant (*Catharanthus roseus*)
- Binds to β-tubulin, which prevents polymerization and therefore inhibits microtubule assembly/promotes disassembly (reminder: taxanes prevent the disassembly of microtubules)
- Cell cycle specific to the G2/M phase
- Liposomal vincristine is a sphingomyelin/cholesterol liposome–encapsulated formulation of vincristine sulfate

What are the common mechanisms of resistance to vinca alkaloid therapy?

- Overexpression of the mdr-1 gene, which encodes for a membrane P-gp efflux pump
- Alterations in the α- and β-tubulin subunits

What are the common dosing ranges for each vinca alkaloid?

- Vincristine: 1.4 mg/m^2 (capped at 2 mg; exception EPOCH)
- Liposomal vincristine: 2.25 mg/m^2 IV over 1 hour once every 7 days (no cap)
- Vinblastine: 4 to 7.4 mg/m^2 every 7 to 14 days
- Vinorelbine: 20 to 30 mg/m^2 every 7 days

Are the vinca alkaloids metabolized/eliminated renally or hepatically?

- All four are extensively metabolized hepatically
- All four vinca alkaloids do not appear to require dose adjustments for renal dysfunction

Are there drug interactions with any of the vinca alkaloids?

- Vincristine and liposomal vincristine: CYP3A4 and P-gp inhibitors/inducers
- Vinblastine: CYP3A4, CYP2D6, and P-gp inhibitors/inducers
- Vinorelbine: CYP3A4 and CYP2D6 inhibitors/inducers

What are the most common adverse effects of each vinca alkaloid?

- Vincristine and liposomal vincristine: constipation, ileus, loss of deep tendon reflex, peripheral neuropathy, jaw pain, syndrome of inappropriate antidiuretic hormone secretion (SIADH)
- Vinblastine: myelosuppression, alopecia, hypertension (due to autonomic dysfunction), malaise, SIADH, less peripheral neuropathy

- Vinorelbine: myelosuppression, granulocytopenia, peripheral neuropathy, constipation, aspartate transaminase (AST)/alanine transaminase (ALT) elevation, alopecia, SIADH, less peripheral neuropathy than vincristine but more than vinblastine

What is the emetogenicity level of the vinca alkaloids?

- All four agents are categorized as low

Are the vinca alkaloids vesicants or irritants?

- All four are vesicants

Alkylating Agents

NITROGEN MUSTARDS

What are the chemotherapy agents in the nitrogen mustard class?

- Mechlorethamine (Mustargen®)
- Cyclophosphamide (Cytoxan®)
- Ifosfamide (Ifex®)
- Bendamustine (Treanda®)
- Chlorambucil (Leukeran®)
- Melphalan (Alkeran®)

What malignancies are each agent FDA approved for?

FDA-Approved Uses of Nitrogen Mustard Alkylating Agents

Agent	FDA Approval
Mechlor-ethamine	Chronic lymphocytic leukemia (CLL), chronic myeloid leukemia (CML), Hodgkin's lymphoma (HL), lymphosarcoma, mycosis fungoides, polycythemia vera, squamous cell carcinoma of the bronchus
Cyclophos-phamide	Acute lymphoblastic leukemia (ALL), acute myeloid leukemia (AML), breast cancer, Burkitt's lymphoma, CLL, CML, HL, malignant histiocytosis, malignant lymphoma—mixed small and large cell, malignant lymphoma—small lymphocytic, mantle cell lymphoma, multiple myeloma (MM), mycosis fungoides, neuroblastoma (disseminated disease), non-Hodgkin's lymphoma (NHL)

(*continued*)

FDA-Approved Uses of Nitrogen Mustard Alkylating Agents (*continued*)

Agent	FDA Approval
Ifosfamide	Testicular cancer (germ cell tumor)
Bendamustine	CLL, NHL (indolent B cell)
Chlorambucil	CLL, HL, mycosis fungoides, NHL
Melphalan	Ovarian cancer (unresectable/palliative), MM

Abbreviation: FDA, U.S. Food and Drug Administration.

How do the nitrogen mustards work?

- Summary: Form cross-links with DNA, inhibiting DNA replication and causing apoptosis

- Nitrogen mustards form reactive, positively charged aziridinium rings by loss of a chloride ion (Figure 2.1). The aziridinium ring then reacts with the nucleophilic centers on DNA (most commonly N-7 of guanine) to form the initial alkylated product. A second aziridinium ring is then formed, which binds to another DNA base, producing a DNA cross-link

- Cyclophosphamide and ifosfamide are prodrugs that are activated to their active metabolites via CYP450 enzymes in the liver

- Bendamustine causes extensive, durable DNA damage due to additional effects on mitotic checkpoints and DNA repair pathways. It is has also been hypothesized that the benzimidazole ring may act as a purine analogue and function as an antimetabolite (Figure 2.2), although this has yet to be proven clinically

- Cross-linking via nitrogen mustards is primarily interstrand

- Cell cycle nonspecific

What are the common mechanisms of resistance to nitrogen mustard therapy?

- Reduced cellular uptake of the drug. Melphalan uptake is dependent on transport via the choline transport system and melphalan is transported via amino acid transport systems. High levels of amino acids, such as leucine, can compete with melphalan for active transport into malignant cells

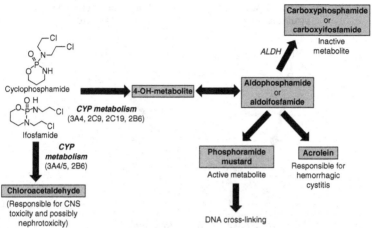

FIGURE 2.1. Cyclophosphamide and ifosfamide metabolic pathway:
Both cyclophosphamide and ifosfamide act as prodrugs and are
metabolized via CYP enzymes to a 4-OH-metabolite. This exists as
a tautomer with the aldophosphamide form. The aldophosphamide
metabolite either is metabolized via aldehyde dehydrogenase (ALDH) to
the inactive carboxy metabolites or undergoes spontaneous breakdown
in cells to the active metabolite phosphoramide mustard and the acrolein
metabolite, which is responsible for hemorrhagic cystitis. Mercaptoethane
sulfonate (mesna) is used to inactivate the acrolein metabolite and prevent
bladder irritation and hemorrhagic cystitis. Of note, CYP enzymes also
convert cyclophosphamide and ifosfamide to the chloroacetaldehyde
metabolite, which is thought to be responsible for central nervous system
(CNS) toxicity as well as potential nephrotoxicity.

- Inactivation of alkylating agents via increased expression of glutathione and glutathione S-transferase

- Increased expression of aldehyde dehydrogenase (ALDH) within malignant cells may increase the conversion of cyclophosphamide and ifosfamide to inactive carboxy metabolites (Figure 2.1)

- Enhanced DNA repair pathways including nucleotide excision repair (NER) and homologous recombination repair

- Defective cell checkpoint function and apoptotic pathways in response to DNA damage

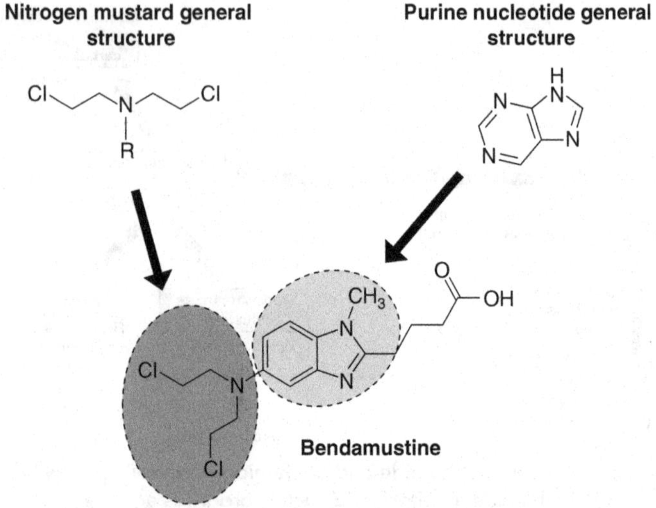

Nitrogen mustard general structure

Purine nucleotide general structure

Bendamustine

FIGURE 2.2. Bendamustine structure: Bendamustine contains a mechlorethamine group that is responsible for its nitrogen mustard alkylating agent activity as well as a benzimidazole ring that mimics the structure of purine analogues, and has been theorized to act as an antimetabolite.

– Loss of mismatch repair (MMR) proteins, which initiate apoptosis

– Loss of normal p53 function

– Upregulation of antiapoptotic proteins (eg, BCL-2, BCL-X$_L$)

What are the common dosing ranges for each nitrogen mustard?

• Mechlorethamine: 6 mg/m^2 intravenous (IV) on days 1 and 8 q28 days (MOPP regimen for Hodgkin's lymphoma [HL])

• Cyclophosphamide: Wide range of dosing, see common examples in the following text

– CyBORD (multiple myeloma [MM]): 300 mg/m^2 orally (PO) days 1, 8, 15, and 22 of a 28-day cycle

– AC (breast cancer): 600 mg/m^2 IV day 1 q21 days

- CHOP (lymphoma): 750 mg/m² IV day 1 q21 days

- CALGB8811 (acute lymphoblastic leukemia [ALL]): 1,200 mg/m² IV day 1 of a 28-day cycle

- HyperCVAD (ALL, lymphoma): 300 mg/m² IV q12h days 1 to 3

- Ifosfamide:

- ICE (lymphoma): 5 g/m² IV continuous infusion day 2 of a 14- to 21-day cycle

- Sarcoma, lymphoma, testicular (several different regimens): 1 to 3 g/m² IV × 3 to 5 days

- Bendamustine: 70 to 120 mg/m² days 1 and 2 of a 21- to 28-day cycle

- Chlorambucil: 0.1 to 0.2 mg/kg PO daily × 3 to 6 weeks; larger doses may be given less frequently (ex: 0.5 mg/kg PO every 2 weeks)

- Melphalan:

- MM (with prednisone): 4 to 6 mg/m²/day for 7 days every 4 weeks

- MM (conditioning for autologous stem cell transplant): 140 to 200 mg/m² IV × 1

Are nitrogen mustards metabolized/eliminated renally or hepatically?

- Cyclophosphamide and ifosfamide are prodrugs, which are metabolized via CYP450 enzymes (2B6, 2C9, 2C19, 3A4) to active metabolites. Both drugs are eliminated renally (mostly as metabolites, including active metabolites and the acrolein metabolite responsible for hemorrhagic cystitis)

- Hepatic dysfunction may decrease production of active phosphoramide mustard metabolites, potentially decreasing efficacy

- Ifosfamide requires dosage adjustment for renal dysfunction; cyclophosphamide may be used safely in cases of renal dysfunction, although caution should be exercised in patients with severe renal impairment

- Chlorambucil and bendamustine are metabolized hepatically. Bendamustine possesses two active metabolites (formed via CYP1A2 metabolism), although metabolite concentrations are significantly lower in plasma than parent drug, indicating only a minor contribution to the cytotoxic activity of bendamustine

- Melphalan undergoes chemical hydrolysis. A small component is eliminated unchanged in urine; thus, in high doses, dosage adjustment may be required for renal impairment

- Mechlorethamine undergoes rapid inactivation in the plasma via hydrolysis

Are there drug interactions with any of the nitrogen mustards?

- Cyclophosphamide/ifosfamide: CYP450 inducers (eg, carbamazepine, phenytoin, rifampin) may increase the production of active metabolites and enhance toxicity. CYP450 inhibitors (eg, azole antifungals, amiodarone, clarithromycin) may decrease the production of active metabolites and compromise efficacy.

- Use of aprepitant/fosaprepitant: may enhance the risk of neurotoxicity with ifosfamide via CYP induction. Because aprepitant and fosaprepitant are also CYP inhibitors, efficacy of cyclophosphamide/ifosfamide may also be compromised.

- Bendamustine: allopurinol may increase the risk of skin reactions with bendamustine, including rash, Stevens-Johnson syndrome, and toxic epidermal necrolysis. Inhibitors or inducers of CYP1A2 will alter the production of active minor metabolites of bendamustine. The clinical impact of this interaction is unknown.

What are the class adverse effects of the nitrogen mustards?

- Myelosuppression
- Nausea/vomiting
- Infertility (depends on dose and agent used)
- Mucositis
- Secondary malignancies:
  - Treatment-related acute myeloid leukemia (AML) is typically associated with deletions in chromosome 5 or 7 and usually occurs 4 to 7 years after exposure

What unique side effects are present with each nitrogen mustard?

- Cyclophosphamide:
  - Hemorrhagic cystitis (more common with higher doses)

– Syndrome of inappropriate antidiuretic hormone (SIADH; more common with higher doses)

– Cardiotoxicity (serious hemorrhagic myocarditis, which is infrequent and seen at higher doses for stem cell transplant)

• Ifosfamide:

– Neurotoxicity/encephalopathy (wide spectrum of signs and symptoms, including sedation, confusion, hallucinations, cerebellar symptoms, seizures, and coma)

– Hemorrhagic cystitis (more common than cyclophosphamide at equivalent doses)

– Renal impairment

• Bendamustine and chlorambucil: skin rashes, hypersensitivity reactions

• Melphalan:

– Mucositis with high doses (conditioning for autologous stem cell transplant; can use ice chips during infusion to lower the risk of severe mucositis)

– SIADH

What are the premedications required?

• Cyclophosphamide/ifosfamide: mercaptoethane sulfonate (mesna)—dose varies depending on regimen

– Continuous infusion (typically 100% of ifosfamide/cyclophosphamide dose)

– Intermittent dosing (60%–100% of ifosfamide/cyclophosphamide dose given with/prior to dose, and 4 and 8 hours after dose)

– When using oral mesna, dose should be doubled to account for approximately 50% bioavailability

What is the emetogenicity level of the nitrogen mustards?

• High: cyclophosphamide ($\geq 1,500$ mg/m^2), mechlorethamine

• Moderate: cyclophosphamide ($<1,500$ mg/m^2), ifosfamide, melphalan, bendamustine

• Minimal: chlorambucil

Are the nitrogen mustards vesicants or irritants?

- Vesicant: mechlorethamine
- Irritant: bendamustine, melphalan, ifosfamide

NON-NITROGEN MUSTARDS

What are the chemotherapy agents in the non-nitrogen mustard alkylating agent class?

Alkyl alkane sulfonates

- Busulfan (Busulfex®, Myleran®)

Nitrosoureas

- Carmustine (BCNU, BiCNU®, Gliadel®)
- Lomustine (CCNU, CeeNU®)
- Streptozocin (Zanosar®)

Aziridines

- Altretamine (Hexalen®)
- Thiotepa (Tepadina®)

Methylating agents

- Dacarbazine (DTIC-Dome®)
- Procarbazine (Matulane®)
- Temozolomide (Temodar®)

What malignancies are each agent FDA approved for?

FDA-Approved Uses of Non-Nitrogen Mustard Alkylating Agents

Agent	FDA Approval
Busulfan	Chronic myeloid leukemia (CML)
Carmustine	Brain tumors, multiple myeloma, Hodgkin's lymphoma (HL; relapsed/refractory), non-Hodgkin's lymphomas (NHL; relapsed/refractory)
Lomustine	Brain tumors, HL (relapsed/refractory)
Streptozocin	Metastatic islet cell carcinoma of the pancreas
Altretamine	Ovarian cancer (persistent/recurrent)

(continued)

FDA-Approved Uses of Non-Nitrogen Mustard Alkylating Agents (*continued*)

Agent	FDA Approval
Thiotepa	Bladder cancer, breast cancer, ovarian cancer, intracavitary effusions due to metastatic tumors
Dacarbazine	Malignant melanoma, HL
Procarbazine	HL
Temozolomide	Anaplastic astrocytoma (refractory), glioblastoma multiforme (newly diagnosed)

Abbreviation: FDA, U.S. Food and Drug Administration.

How do the alkylating agents work?

• Summary: form cross-links with DNA, inhibiting DNA replication and causing apoptosis

• Alkylating agents form reactive intermediates that react with nucleophilic centers on DNA (most commonly N-7 of guanine) but also may bind to proteins, amino acids, and nucleotides

• Alkylating agents with two reactive groups (bifunctional alkylating agents) form DNA cross-links

– Streptozocin is a nitrosourea that contains a glucose moiety, which may explain its selectivity toward pancreatic beta cells

• Methylating agents (procarbazine, dacarbazine, temozolomide) transfer a single methyl group to DNA bases

– Procarbazine and dacarbazine primarily create O-6 methylguanine adducts. Temozolomide primarily methylates N–7 of guanine; adducts to the O-6 of guanine are critical for cytotoxicity

– Procarbazine and dacarbazine are metabolized in the liver to active metabolites. Temozolomide spontaneously converts to its active metabolite [3-methyl-(triazen-1-yl)imidazole-4-carboxamide—MTIC] in aqueous solution

• DNA cross-linking and alkylation inhibits DNA synthesis. Attempts at repair of DNA alkylation and cross-linking lead to DNA strand breakage

• Cell cycle checkpoint proteins recognize the DNA damage, halt cell cycle progression, and initiate apoptosis

- Cross-linking with bifunctional alkylating agents is primarily inter-strand
- Cell cycle nonspecific

What are the common mechanisms of resistance to alkylating agent therapy?

- Inactivation of alkylating agents via increased expression of glutathione and glutathione S-transferase
- Enhanced DNA repair pathways, including base excision repair, enzymes that catalyze the removal of alkyl groups from guanine bases (alkylguanine-O^6-alkyltransferase [AGT], encoded by the O^6-methylguanine methyltransferase [MGMT] gene), NER, and homologous recombination repair

  – Lower AGT levels due to methylation of the promoter region of the MGMT gene lead to enhanced sensitivity of tumors to alkylating agents (eg, improved survival of glioblastoma patients with methylated MGMT promoters receiving temozolomide and radiation therapy)

  – AGT is the primary mechanism of resistance to the methylating agents temozolomide, procarbazine, and dacarbazine, and this enzyme contributes resistance to lomustine and carmustine as well

- Defective cell checkpoint function and apoptotic pathways in response to DNA damage

  – Induction of the Akt signaling pathway, which inhibits apoptotic pathways

  – Loss of MMR proteins, which initiate apoptosis

  – Loss of normal p53 function

  – Upregulation of antiapoptotic proteins (eg, BCL-2, BCL-X_L)

What are the common dosing ranges for each alkylating agent?

- Busulfan:

  – 3.2 to 4 mg/kg/day IV (may be given in divided dosing) $\times$ 2 to 4 days (bone marrow transplant [BMT] conditioning)

  – 1 to 8 mg/day PO (chronic myeloid leukemia [CML], essential thrombocythemia [ET], polycythemia vera [PV])

- Carmustine:
  - 150 to 200 mg/m^2 IV q6–8 weeks (may be given over 2 days)
  - Autologous hematopoietic stem cell transplantation (HSCT): 300 to 600 mg/m^2 prior to transplant (eg, BEAM, CBV regimens)
  - Glioblastoma multiforme: Up to eight wafers (61.6 mg) in resection cavity
- Lomustine: 100 to 130 mg/m^2 PO × 1 q6 weeks
- Streptozocin:
  - 500 mg/m^2/day × 5 days q6 weeks
  - 1,000 to 1,500 mg/m^2 once weekly
- Altretamine:
  - 260 mg/m^2 daily in four divided doses × 14 to 21 days of a 28-day cycle
- Thiotepa:
  - BMT conditioning: 250 mg/m^2/day × 3 days or 150 mg/m^2 q12h × 6 doses
  - Ovarian/breast cancer: 0.3 to 0.4 mg/kg q1–4 weeks
  - Intravesicular: 60 mg in 30 to 60 mL normal saline (NS) retained for 2 hours weekly × 4 weeks
  - Intrathecal (leptomeningeal metastases): 10 mg twice a week (days 1 and 4) × 8 weeks
- Dacarbazine:
  - ABVD: 375 mg/m^2 days 1 and 15 q28 days
  - Metastatic melanoma: 250 mg/m^2/dose days 1 to 5 q3 weeks or 1,000 mg/m^2 IV every 3 to 4 weeks
- Procarbazine: 60 to 100 mg/m^2 PO × 7 to 14 days
- Temozolomide:
  - Glioblastoma (newly diagnosed, concomitant radiotherapy): 75 mg/m^2 PO daily × 42 days
  - 150 mg/m^2 PO daily × 5 days every 28 days (increase to 200 mg/m^2 next cycle if nadir blood counts acceptable)

Are alkylating agents metabolized/eliminated renally or hepatically?

- Busulfan: Extensively hepatically metabolized; dose adjust for hepatic dysfunction

- Carmustine: Metabolized hepatically to active metabolites and excreted in the urine; dose adjust for renal dysfunction and severe hepatic dysfunction

- Lomustine: Metabolized hepatically to active metabolites and excreted in the urine; dose adjust for renal dysfunction and severe hepatic dysfunction

- Streptozocin: Metabolized hepatically and excreted in the urine; dose adjust for renal dysfunction and severe hepatic dysfunction

- Altretamine: Metabolized hepatically to active metabolites and excreted in the urine; dose adjust for renal dysfunction and severe hepatic dysfunction

- Thiotepa: Metabolized hepatically to active and inactive metabolites and excreted in the urine; dose adjust for renal and severe hepatic dysfunction

- Dacarbazine: Hepatically metabolized to active metabolites and excreted in the urine; dose adjust for renal dysfunction and/or severe hepatic dysfunction

- Procarbazine: Hepatically oxidized to active metabolites (further metabolized to inactive metabolites); dose adjust for hepatic dysfunction

- Temozolomide: Eliminated renally; dose adjust for severe renal dysfunction

Are there drug interactions with any of the alkylating agents?

- Procarbazine inhibits monoamine oxidase (MAO); avoid tyramine-containing foods, sympathomimetics (eg, dopamine), tricyclic antidepressants, other serotonin and norepinephrine concentration modifying drugs (selective serotonin reuptake inhibitors [SSRIs], serotonin–norepinephrine reuptake inhibitors [SNRIs], linezolid), and other MAO inhibitors to prevent risk of hypertensive crisis and serotonin syndrome

• Procarbazine may produce a disulfiram-like reaction when taken with alcohol

• Procarbazine/dacarbazine: Metabolized via CYP enzymes to active metabolite. CYP450 inducers (eg, carbamazepine, phenytoin, rifampin) may increase the production of active metabolites and enhance toxicity. CYP450 inhibitors (eg, azole antifungals, amiodarone, clarithromycin) may decrease the production of active metabolites and compromise efficacy

• Busulfan is metabolized primarily by conjugation via glutathione S-transferase and partially via CYP450 metabolism. Interactions resulting in increased busulfan concentrations have been reported with azole antifungals (itraconazole), acetaminophen, metronidazole, phenytoin, and phenytoin. Phenytoin concentrations should also be monitored in patients receiving busulfan, as reductions in phenytoin levels have been observed

 – Although the IV formulation has improved delivery of busulfan, due to variability in busulfan pharmacokinetics, first-dose therapeutic drug monitoring may be useful in select patients

• Cimetidine has been reported to enhance myelosuppression due to carmustine and lomustine (mechanism unknown)

• Altretamine used in combination with MAO inhibitors increases the risk of severe orthostatic hypotension

What are the class adverse effects of the alkylating agents?

• Myelosuppression

• Nausea/vomiting

• Infertility (depends on dose and agent used)

• Secondary malignancies

 – Treatment-related AML is typically associated with deletions in chromosome 5 or 7 and usually occurs 4 to 7 years after exposure

What unique side effects are present with each alkylating agent?

• Procarbazine: hemolysis (in G6PD-deficient patients), neurotoxicity (central nervous system [CNS] depression—avoid other CNS-depressing agents—dizziness, drowsiness, confusion), hypersensitivity reactions (rash, pneumonitis [rarely])

• Dacarbazine: flulike syndrome (fevers, chills, myalgias for several days after therapy), photosensitivity

• Temozolomide: myelosuppression (primarily lymphopenia—prophylaxis for *Pneumocystis* pneumonia (PCP) should be initiated for those receiving concomitant temozolomide and radiation therapy and in those who become lymphopenic)

• Busulfan: mucositis, skin hyperpigmentation and rash, alopecia, pulmonary fibrosis ("busulfan lung"), hepatotoxicity (veno-occlusive disease [VOD]), neurotoxicity (CNS depression, anxiety, headache, confusion, dizziness, seizures; use prophylactic anticonvulsants when using for BMT conditioning)

• Carmustine: mucositis, pulmonary fibrosis (risk increases at cumulative doses >1,400 mg/m^2), hepatotoxicity (VOD), neurotoxicity (ataxia, dizziness, headache), alcohol intoxication with high doses (formulated with ethanol), facial flushing, skin irritation and injection site pain, hypotension (infuse over >2 hours to minimize injection site pain, flushing, and hypotension), skin hyperpigmentation and pain (after skin contact), alopecia

• Lomustine: pulmonary fibrosis (uncommon at doses <1,100 mg/m^2), neurotoxicity (confusion, ataxia, lethargy, disorientation), nephrotoxicity

• Streptozocin: hyperglycemia/glucose intolerance (due to pancreatic beta cell toxicity), nephrotoxicity, pain/irritation at injection site, liver function test (LFT) elevations (usually transient)

• Altretamine: peripheral sensory neuropathy, neurotoxicity (mood disturbances, somnolence, agitation, depression, dizziness)

• Thiotepa: mucositis, alopecia, dermatologic changes (dermatitis, erythema, pruritus, pigmentation changes), hepatotoxicity (VOD), neurotoxicity (dizziness, headache, seizures, confusion), hypersensitivity reactions, pneumonitis

What are the premedications required?

• Busulfan: prophylactic anticonvulsants should be utilized with BMT (seizures usually occur during administration or within 24 to 48 hours after the last dose)

• All other non-nitrogen mustard alkylating agents do not require premedications

What is the emetogenicity level of the alkylating agents?

• High: procarbazine, dacarbazine, carmustine (>250 mg/m^2), streptozocin, altretamine, thiotepa (≥ 300 mg/m^2 in children)

• Moderate: temozolomide, busulfan, carmustine (≤ 250 mg/m^2), lomustine, thiotepa (adults; <300 mg/m^2 in children)

Are the alkylating agents vesicants or irritants?

• Dacarbazine, busulfan, carmustine, and streptozocin are irritants

• All other agents are neither vesicants nor irritants

PLATINUMS

What are the chemotherapy agents in the platinum class?

- Cisplatin (Platinol®)
- Carboplatin (Paraplatin®)
- Oxaliplatin (Eloxatin®)

What malignancies are each platinum FDA approved for?

FDA-Approved Uses of Platinum Alkylating Agents

Agent	FDA Approval
Cisplatin	Advanced bladder cancer, metastatic testicular cancer, metastatic ovarian cancer
Carboplatin	Advanced ovarian cancer
Oxaliplatin	Stage III colon cancer, advanced colorectal cancer

Abbreviation: FDA, U.S. Food and Drug Administration.

How do the platinums work? (See Figure 2.3)

- Form cross-links between purine nucleosides (guanine and adenine) of DNA (~95% intrastrand), causing DNA kinking, interference with normal DNA function, and ultimately cell death

- Cross-linking of DNA triggers DNA repair via the NER pathway and double-strand break repair process. When DNA cross-links are not effectively repaired, cell death occurs

- May also bind RNA and various cellular proteins; however, majority of cytotoxicity thought to be related to DNA intrastrand cross-links

- Binding to nuclear and cytoplasmic proteins may result in cytotoxic effects

- Synergistic with radiation (a radiosensitizer) and other DNA-damaging agents

- Cell cycle–nonspecific agent

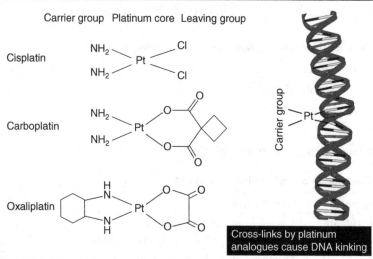

Cross-links by platinum analogues cause DNA kinking

FIGURE 2.3. Platinum structure and mechanism of action.

What are the common mechanisms of resistance to platinum therapy?

• Increased activity of DNA repair pathways (eg, NER)

• Inactivation of drug by binding to sulfhydryl groups on cytosolic proteins (eg, glutathione)

• Reduced uptake into or active efflux out of cells via copper transport pathways (CTR1, ATP7A, ATP7B)

• Decreased apoptosis in response to DNA damage

  – Loss of MMR proteins, which initiate apoptosis

What are the common dosing ranges for each platinum?

• Cisplatin: 50 to 100 mg/m² every 3 to 4 weeks

• Carboplatin: Use Calvert equation to calculate dose (usual area under the curve [AUC] 5–6). If estimating glomerular filtration rate (GFR), FDA recommends considering capping GFR at 125 mL/min

  – Dose = Target AUC (GFR + 25)

• Oxaliplatin: 85 to 130 mg/m² every 2 to 3 weeks

Are the platinums metabolized/eliminated renally or hepatically?

- Platinums are eliminated via the kidney and require dose adjustments
  - Carboplatin is dosed via GFR and the Calvert equation
- Platinums do not require dosage adjustment for hepatic dysfunction

Are there drug interactions with the platinums?

Platinums should be administered after taxane derivatives to limit myelosuppression and enhance efficacy

- Cisplatin/carboplatin—concomitant nephrotoxic drugs, IV thiosulfates may inactivate drug, phenytoin, lithium (due to cation wasting with nephrotoxicity)
- Oxaliplatin—synergistic with 5-fluorouracil (5-FU), must be prepared in dextrose solutions (other platinums are stabilized by NS)

What are the class adverse effects of the platinums?

- Nephrotoxicity—cisplatin > carboplatin > oxaliplatin
- Nausea/vomiting—cisplatin > carboplatin/oxaliplatin
- Neuropathy
- Myelosuppression—carboplatin > cisplatin > oxaliplatin
- Acute hypersensitivity (usually occurs after 6th–8th exposure to the drug)

What are the most common adverse effects of each platinum?

- Cisplatin—Nausea/vomiting (highly emetogenic), nephrotoxicity with cation wasting (hypomagnesemia, hypokalemia, hypocalcemia), myelosuppression (more thrombocytopenia), ototoxicity (high tone loss), peripheral neuropathy, hypersensitivity
- Carboplatin—Myelosuppression (more thrombocytopenia and neutropenia), nausea/vomiting (moderate), nephrotoxicity, peripheral neuropathy, hypersensitivity

• Oxaliplatin—Acute neuropathy (usually within 7 days) commonly triggered by cold exposure (patients should avoid cold beverages/ foods to prevent laryngopharyngeal dysesthesia), cumulative and chronic neuropathy, nausea/vomiting (moderate), myelosuppression (less than other platinums—likely related to concomitant 5-FU use), and hepatotoxicity

What are the premedications required?

• Premedications (other than antiemetics) are generally not required for platinum derivatives

• Prior to cisplatin administration, hydration with 1 to 2 L of fluid is recommended; adequate hydration should be maintained for 24 hours after administration

• Do not give ice chips or cold beverages/foods during (or within 7 days) of oxaliplatin infusion

What is the emetogenicity level of the platinums?

• Cisplatin—high
• Carboplatin/oxaliplatin—moderate

Are the platinums vesicants or irritants?

• Platinums are classified as irritants

ANTITUMOR ANTIBIOTICS

What are the chemotherapy agents in this class?

- Bleomycin (Blenoxane®)
- Dactinomycin (Cosmegen®, actinomycin D)
- Mitomycin C (Mutamycin®, MMC)—*Streptomyces caespitosus*

What malignancies are the antitumor antibiotics FDA approved for?

FDA-Approved Uses of Antitumor Antibiotics

Agent	FDA Approval
Bleomycin	Head and neck cancers, Hodgkin's lymphoma, malignant pleural effusions, testicular and other germ cell tumors
Dactinomycin	Choriocarcinoma, pediatric sarcomas, Wilms' tumor, neuroblastoma, rhabdomyosarcoma, and Ewing sarcoma
Mitomycin	Anal carcinomas and bladder instillation in bladder cancer

Abbreviation: FDA, U.S. Food and Drug Administration.

How do the antitumor antibiotics work?

- Bleomycin: A_2 peptide
  - Generates free radicals by binding to Fe, causing single and double DNA strand breaks
    - Oxygen binds to iron leading to the formation of Fe(II)-bleomycin-O_2
    - The complex binds in the minor groove to guanosine-cytosine–rich portions of DNA by forming an "S" tripeptide and partial intercalation of the bithiazole rings. This will stabilize the Fe(II)-bleomycin-O_2 complex. In the absence of DNA, the complex will self-destruct

- Reactive oxygen species (ROS) will cause double and single DNA strand breaks
- Inhibits RNA and protein synthesis to a lesser degree

- Dactinomycin
  - Intercalation of double-stranded DNA by chromophore of dactinomycin, inserts between the guanine-cytidine base pairs
  - Binds to single-stranded DNA, prevents reannealing of DNA, and stabilizes unusual hairpins resulting in inhibition of transcription

- Mitomycin
  - Forms DNA adducts by cross-linking complementary double-stranded and single-stranded DNA (alkylator) → inhibits DNA replication
    - Binds different parts of guanine depending on the way it formed a ROS
  - Anaerobic: Undergoes reduction reaction to form reactive unstable intermediates, which forms a covalent monoadduct with DNA
  - Aerobic: DT-diaphorase (DTD) enzyme and nicotinamide adenine dinucleotide phosphate (NADPH) metabolize MMC to reactive cytotoxic species (prodrug)

What are common mechanisms of resistance to each agent?

- Bleomycin: bleomycin hydrolase enzyme hydrolyzes terminal amine, inhibiting the iron-binding capacity (and cytotoxic activity) of the drug
  - Enzyme protects normal tissue, but is in low concentration in the skin and lungs
- Dactinomycin: efflux by P170 glycoprotein pump encoded by the MDR gene
- Mitomycin: loss of MMC activation capacity, increased DNA repair mechanisms, P170 efflux pump

What are the common dosing ranges for each agent?

- Bleomycin
  - HL

- ○ ABVD: 10 units/m^2 on days 1 and 15 of each 28-day cycle
- ○ BEACOPP: 10 units/m^2 on day 8 of each 21-day cycle
- ○ Stanford 5: 5 units/m^2 weeks 2, 4, 6, 8, 10, and 12

– Testicular cancer and other germ cell tumors, BEP: 30 units/week × 12 doses

– Intrapleural or intraperitoneal injections for malignant effusions to breast, lung, and ovarian cancers: 60 units/m^2 in 50 to 100 mL of NS

• Dactinomycin

– Pediatric dosing: 12 to 15 mcg/kg/day × 5 days each cycle

– Adult dosing: 300 to 600 mcg/m^2/day × 5 days each cycle

• Mitomycin

– Stomach and pancreas adenocarcinoma: 20 mg/m^2 every 6 to 8 weeks

– Anal carcinoma: 10 mg/m^2 every 4 weeks

– Intravesicular instillation for bladder cancer: 40-mg dose × 1 or 20 mg weekly × 6 weeks, then monthly for 3 years

Are the agents metabolized/eliminated renally or hepatically?

• Bleomycin: renal
• Dactinomycin: renal and biliary
• Mitomycin: hepatic metabolism, renal elimination

Are there drug interactions with any of the agents?

• Bleomycin

a. Will form complexes with copper, cobalt, iron, zinc, and manganese

b. Cisplatin decreases bleomycin clearance

c. Radiation therapy produces additive free radical damage to DNA resulting in additive pulmonary toxicity

d. Brentuximab and filgrastim/pegfilgrastim can increase lung toxicity when given with bleomycin

• Dactinomycin: radiosensitizer
• Mitomycin: radiosensitizer

What are the adverse effects of each agent?

- Bleomycin: Thrombophlebitis, rash, blisters, hyperkeratosis, hyperpigmentation, fevers, hypersensitivities (chills, fever, anaphylaxis; test dose not predictive), pulmonary dysfunction (pneumonitis, fibrosis), Raynaud's disease, very low likelihood for myelosuppression

  a. Pulmonary fibrosis (dose-limiting toxicity [DLT], cumulative above 400 units)

    i. Develops slowly; usually presents as pneumonitis with cough, dyspnea, dry inspiratory crackles, and chest x-ray infiltrates

    ii. Causes direct inflammatory response, epithelial apoptosis, and progressive deposition of collagen over 1 to 2 weeks → pulmonary fibrosis

    iii. Increased risk with age >70 (>40 for germ cell tumor patients), underlying pulmonary dysfunction, or chest radiation therapy, decreased renal function, growth factors (filgrastim/pegfilgrastim), single doses >25 units/m^2

    iv. Due to lack of bleomycin hydrolase in lung

    v. Associated with single high doses versus smaller daily doses

- Dactinomycin: Myelosuppression (DLT), nausea/vomiting, diarrhea, alopecia, rare VOD, radiation recall, interstitial pneumonitis

- Mitomycin: Gastrointestinal (GI) side effects are mild and infrequent, hemolytic uremic syndrome, interstitial pneumonitis, cardiomyopathy, rare VOD

  a. Myelosuppression

    i. Common with low daily doses, less common with boluses every 4 to 8 weeks

    ii. Rare <50 mg/m^2; at higher doses, thrombocytopenia is more common than anemia and leukocytopenia

What are the premedications required?

- Bleomycin: some investigators advocate for test doses for lymphoma patients due to rare instances of allergic reactions

- Antiemetics

What is the emetogenicity level of the antitumor antibiotics?

- Bleomycin: minimal
- Dactinomycin: moderate
- Mitomycin: low

Are the antitumor antibiotics vesicants or irritants?

- Bleomycin: nonvesicant, nonirritant
- Dactinomycin: vesicant—requires cold compress
- Mitomycin: vesicant—requires cold compress and dimethyl sulfoxide (DMSO)

Enzyme Inhibitors—Topoisomerase I Inhibitors

What are the chemotherapy agents in the topoisomerase I inhibitor class?

- Irinotecan (Camptosar®) and topotecan (Hycamtin®)

What malignancies are the topoisomerase I inhibitors approved for by the U.S. Food and Drug Administration (FDA)?

FDA-Approved Uses of Topoisomerase I Inhibitors

Agent	FDA Approval
Irinotecan	Metastatic colorectal cancer
Topotecan	Cervical cancer, metastatic ovarian cancer, small cell lung cancer

Abbreviation: FDA, U.S. Food and Drug Administration.

How do the topoisomerase I inhibitors work?

- Topoisomerase I is an enzyme that relieves tension and supercoiling of DNA by binding to DNA and creating transient single-strand breaks, forming what is known as the cleavable complex

- Topoisomerase I inhibitors bind to the enzyme and stabilize the normally transient cleavable complex and prevent religation of DNA

- Collision of the DNA replication fork with the cleavable complex prevents DNA replication and produces DNA strand breaks, leading to apoptosis. Accumulation of supercoils ahead of the replication fork also contributes to cytotoxicity

- Irinotecan is a prodrug that must be converted to its active metabolite, SN-38, via a carboxylesterase enzyme (Figure 3.1)

- Cell cycle phase specific (S phase)

What are the common mechanisms of resistance to topoisomerase inhibitors?

- Point mutations in topoisomerase I that prevent camptothecin binding

- Alterations in carboxylesterase enzyme concentrations may reduce activation of irinotecan to its active metabolite, SN38 (Figure 3.1)

- Decreased expression of topoisomerase I within tumor cells

- Active efflux and reduced accumulation in tumor cells secondary to active transport mechanisms (P-glycoprotein [P-gp], organic anion-transporting polypeptides [OATPs])

- Altered intracellular localization of topoisomerase I (nucleolus vs. nucleus/cytoplasm), reducing its interaction with DNA and subsequent cellular cytotoxicity in the presence of camptothecins

- Reduced cell death in response to camptothecin/topoisomerase I/DNA complex formation secondary to alterations in DNA damage checkpoint and apoptotic pathways (eg, ERK, BCL-2, Chk-1/Chk-2, MAPK)

What are the common dosing ranges for the topoisomerase I inhibitors?

- Irinotecan (several dosing strategies exist, the most common are in the following text)

- 65 to 125 mg/m^2 intravenous (IV) weekly $\times$ 4 weeks (6-week cycle)

- 165 to 180 mg/m^2 IV every 2 weeks (FOLFIRINOX)

- 250 to 350 mg/m^2 IV every 3 weeks

- Topotecan

  - 0.75 to 1.5 mg/m^2 IV $\times$ 3 to 5 days every 21 days

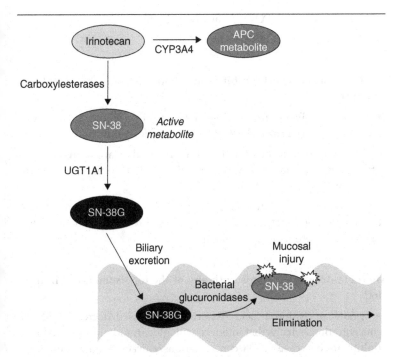

FIGURE 3.1. Irinotecan metabolism and elimination: Irinotecan is converted via carboxylesterases (primarily carboxylesterase 2 in humans) to an active metabolite, SN-38. It also undergoes hepatic oxidation, primarily via CYP3A4, to a 100-fold less-active metabolite, APC. The SN-38 metabolite is responsible for the majority of cytotoxicity of irinotecan. This agent undergoes glucuronidation via several UGT1A isoforms, with UGT1A1 being the most predominant. Polymorphisms exist in the UGT1A1 enzyme, and patients with UGT1A1*28 alleles have reduced glucuronidation of active SN-38 and are at increased risk for irinotecan toxicities (neutropenia and diarrhea). SN-38G is excreted via the biliary route. Bacterial glucuronidases in the gastrointestinal (GI) tract convert SN-38G back to the active SN-38, and this may be responsible for the late-onset diarrhea of irinotecan. Several studies have utilized cephalosporin prophylaxis to reduce bacterial conversion of SN-38G to active SN-38 to reduce diarrhea and improve compliance, primarily in pediatric patients.

– 2.3 mg/m^2 orally (PO) × 5 days every 21 days

– 4 mg/m^2 days 1, 8, and 15 every 28 days

Are the topoisomerase I inhibitors metabolized/eliminated renally or hepatically?

- Irinotecan—Primarily eliminated hepatically (Figure 3.1) and excreted via biliary routes; dose adjust for hepatic dysfunction

  – Patients homozygous for the UGT1A1*28 allele are at higher risk for severe neutropenia and may require reduced initial doses of irinotecan

- Topotecan—Primarily renally eliminated (undergoes glucuronidation and minor hepatic metabolism) and requires dose adjustment for moderate/severe renal impairment

Are there drug interactions with any of the topoisomerase I inhibitors?

- Irinotecan—valproic acid (reports of increased/decreased SN-38 concentrations), drugs that interfere with glucuronidation via UGT1A1 (inhibitors decrease SN-38 concentrations/efficacy, inducers increase SN-38 concentrations/toxicity), drugs that affect CYP3A4

- Topotecan—P-gp inhibitors/inducers

What are the class adverse effects of the topoisomerase I inhibitors?

- Myelosuppression (neutropenia predominates), alopecia, mucositis

What are the most common adverse effects of each topoisomerase I inhibitor?

- Irinotecan—early-onset diarrhea (during infusion or within first 12–24 hours), associated with flushing, diaphoresis, and cramping (due to inhibition of acetylcholinesterase activity by irinotecan; treat with atropine), late-onset diarrhea (manage with antidiarrheals; consider cephalosporin use—see Figure 3.1), myelosuppression (primarily neutropenia, less common with weekly administration), nausea/vomiting, increased liver function tests (LFTs), fatigue

- Topotecan—late-onset diarrhea (does not produce cholinergic reaction like irinotecan), mucositis, myelosuppression, fatigue, nausea/vomiting, rash, increased LFTs

What are the premedications required?

- No routine premedications (other than standard antiemetics) required
- Can consider premedication with atropine in patients who experience cholinergic symptoms with irinotecan

What is the emetogenicity level of the topoisomerase I inhibitors?

- Irinotecan and topotecan have a low emetogenic potential

Are the topoisomerase I inhibitors vesicants or irritants?

- Irinotecan and topotecan are irritants

4

Enzyme Inhibitors—Topoisomerase II Inhibitors

EPIPODOPHYLLOTOXINS

What are the chemotherapy agents in the topoisomerase II Inhibitor class?

- The epipodophyllotoxins, etoposide (Toposar®; Vepesid®; VP-16), etoposide phosphate (Etopophos®), and teniposide (Vumon®; VM-26)

  - Etoposide phosphate is a water-soluble prodrug of etoposide that is rapidly and completely converted to etoposide in plasma with equivalent bioavailability

What malignancies are the topoisomerase II inhibitors FDA approved for?

FDA-Approved Uses of Topoisomerase II Inhibitors

Agent	FDA Approval
Etoposide	Small cell lung cancer, testicular cancer (refractory)
Teniposide	Acute lymphoblastic leukemia (ALL) (refractory)

Abbreviation: FDA, U.S. Food and Drug administration.

How do the topoisomerase II inhibitors work?

- Topoisomerase II is an enzyme that relieves tension and supercoiling of DNA by binding to DNA and creating transient double-strand breaks, forming what is known as the cleavable complex

- Epipodophyllotoxins are pure topoisomerase II inhibitors (no free radical formation or DNA intercalation, unlike anthracyclines). These agents bind to the enzyme and stabilize the normally transient cleavable complex, preventing religation of DNA and producing DNA strand breaks

- Epipodophyllotoxins produce a mixture of DNA single- and double-strand breaks (compared to anthracyclines, more single-strand breaks are produced)

- Cell cycle phase specific (S/G_2 phase)

What are the common mechanisms of resistance to topoisomerase II inhibitors?

- Active efflux and reduced drug accumulation in tumor cells due to active transport mechanisms (P-glycoprotein [P-gp], multidrug resistance–associated proteins [MRPs], breast cancer resistance protein [BCRP])

- Reduced drug accumulation in the nucleus, possibly due to nuclear efflux transporters or sequestration in the cytoplasm

- Decreased expression of topoisomerase II within tumor cells

- Altered intracellular localization of topoisomerase II (a shift from the nucleus to the cytoplasm), reducing its interaction with DNA and subsequent cellular cytotoxicity in the presence of topoisomerase II inhibitors

- Alterations in phosphorylation of topoisomerase II (both hypophosphorylation and hyperphosphorylation have been associated with drug resistance)

- Reduced cell death in response to drug-induced DNA damage secondary to alterations in DNA damage checkpoint and apoptotic pathways (eg, B-cell lymphoma 2 [BCL-2])

What are the common dosing ranges for the topoisomerase II inhibitors?

- Etoposide—50 to 100 mg/m^2 intravenous (IV) $\times$ 3 to 5 days q3–4 weeks

  – Note: Oral bioavailability is variable and ranges from approximately 25% to 75%

– Etoposide phosphate is a prodrug of etoposide that is rapidly and completely converted to etoposide in plasma

- Teniposide—165 mg/m^2/dose IV days 1, 4, 8, 11

Are the topoisomerase II inhibitors metabolized/eliminated renally or hepatically?

- Etoposide—metabolized hepatically via CYP3A4/3A5 (some metabolites are active metabolites), as well as through glucuronide (via UGT1A1) and glutathione conjugation. Approximately 50% of a dose is eliminated unchanged in the urine. Dose adjust if both renal and hepatic dysfunction present (renal excretion can compensate for hepatic dysfunction).

  – Because of a high degree of protein binding, dose reductions may be required in the setting of hypoalbuminemia where the unbound fraction of etoposide is higher (eg, in the setting of severe hepatic dysfunction or poor nutritional status).

- Teniposide—primarily eliminated hepatically; dose adjust for hepatic dysfunction.

Are there drug interactions with any of the topoisomerase II inhibitors?

- Drugs that inhibit/induce CYP3A4

- P-gp inhibitors/inducers

- Other highly protein-bound drugs that compete with topoisomerase II inhibitors for albumin protein binding (eg, warfarin, valproic acid, phenytoin)

What are the most common adverse effects of the topoisomerase II inhibitors?

- Myelosuppression (neutropenia predominates), alopecia, mucositis, nausea/vomiting, secondary malignancies (frequently involving MLL gene [found at chromosome band 11q23] rearrangements; latency period is typically shorter [median ~1–2 years] than that expected with alkylating agent–associated malignancies), hypotension associated with more rapid infusion.

• Etoposide and teniposide are formulated with polysorbate 80 and Cremophor® EL, respectively, in addition to containing significant alcohol content (~30%–40% v/v). These excipients may play a role in hypersensitivity reactions, hypotension, and ethanol intoxication side effects (with higher doses used in stem cell transplantation). Etoposide phosphate does not contain these excipients.

What are the premedications required?

• No routine premedications (other than standard antiemetics) required

What is the emetogenicity level of the topoisomerase II inhibitors?

• Etoposide and teniposide have a low emetogenic potential

Are the topoisomerase II inhibitors vesicants or irritants?

• Etoposide and teniposide are irritants

ANTHRACYCLINES

What are the chemotherapy agents in this class?

- Doxorubicin (Adriamycin®), liposomal doxorubicin (Doxil®, Lipodox®)

- Epirubicin (Ellence®)

- Mitoxantrone (Novantrone®)—is an anthracenedione

- Daunorubicin (Cerubidine®), liposomal daunorubicin (DaunoXome®)

- Idarubicin (Idamycin PFS®)

What malignancies are the anthracyclines FDA approved for?

FDA-Approved Uses of Anthracyclines

Agent	FDA Approval
Doxorubicin	Breast cancer Metastatic cancers or disseminated neoplastic conditions: acute myeloid leukemia (AML), acute lymphoblastic leukemia (ALL), Wilms' tumor, neuroblastoma, soft tissue and bone sarcomas, ovarian cancer, transitional cell bladder carcinoma, gastric carcinoma, Hodgkin's lymphoma (HL), non-Hodgkin's lymphoma (NHL), bronchogenic carcinoma, thyroid cancer
Liposomal doxorubicin	Ovarian (2nd line after platinums), multiple myeloma (2nd line with bortezomib), AIDS-related Kaposi's sarcoma
Epirubicin	Breast cancer

(continued)

FDA-Approved Uses of Anthracyclines (*continued*)

Agent	FDA Approval
Mitoxantrone	Acute nonlymphocytic leukemias (myelogenous, promyelocytic, monocytic, erythroid), hormone-refractory prostate cancer
Idarubicin	AML
Daunorubicin	AML and ALL
Liposomal daunorubicin	AIDS-related Kaposi's sarcoma, ovarian cancer, multiple myeloma

Abbreviation: FDA, U.S. Food and Drug administration.

How do the anthracyclines work?

- Complex with DNA and topoisomerase II

    – Topoisomerase II relieves torsional strain by breaking the phosphate backbone of DNA during replication and reannealing it after replication is complete

    – Topoisomerase II–induced strand breaks are potentiated by binding of anthracyclines

    – The binding of anthracyclines also prevents reannealing of the DNA phosphate backbone

- Anthracyclines also may intercalate with DNA

    – Inhibits DNA and RNA synthesis

- Some anthracyclines produce free radicals leading to direct DNA, cell membrane, and mitochondrial damage (doxorubicin has greater free radical production than other anthracyclines)

What are the common mechanisms of resistance to anthracycline therapy?

- MDR1 gene coding for P170 glycoprotein responsible for the efflux of anthracyclines out of a cell

- Other adenosine triphosphate (ATP)-dependent efflux transporters (MRP, BRCP) pump anthracyclines out of tumor cells and into normal host tissue (eg, liver)
- Reduction or absence of topoisomerase II activity
- Overexpression of BCL-2 and mutations of p53
- Increased DNA repair systems

What are the common dosing ranges for each anthracycline?

Anthracyclines have generally equivalent antitumor activity (but different toxicities) whether dosed as a single large monthly bolus, single large weekly bolus, or prolonged infusion

- Doxorubicin
  - Dose-response relationship in solid tumors
  - 40 to 75 mg/m^2 every 3 weeks
  - 25 to 30 mg/m^2 every 7 to 14 days
- Liposomal doxorubicin
  - 20 to 30 mg/m^2 every 21 days
  - 50 mg/m^2 every 28 days
- Epirubicin
  - 100 to 120 mg/m^2 every 21 to 28 days (breast cancer)
  - 60 mg/m^2 every week
- Mitoxantrone
  - 8 to 14 mg/m^2 every 21 to 28 days
  - 6 mg/m$^2 \times$ 6 days (MEC)
- Idarubicin
  - 8 to 12 mg/m$^2 \times$ 3 days
- Daunorubicin
  - 30 to 90 mg/m^2/day $\times$ 3 days

Are the anthraclines metabolized/eliminated renally or hepatically?

- All anthracyclines undergo hepatic metabolism with biliary excretion
- All should be dose adjusted for hepatic dysfunction
- Dose adjustments for renal dysfunction vary in clinical practice

Are there drug interactions with any of the anthracyclines?

- Doxorubicin:
  - Overlapping cardiotoxicity with other agents (bevacizumab, trastuzumab)
  - P-gp, cytochrome P450 3A4 and 2D6 interactions
  - P-gp inducer; inhibits CYP2B6 (moderate), CYP2D6 (weak), CYP3A4 (weak)
  - Taxanes decrease doxorubicin metabolism, but docetaxel has less of an interaction. Administer doxorubicin prior to paclitaxel when used concomitantly
- Liposomal doxorubicin: less cardiotoxicity interactions, otherwise same as conventional form
- Epirubicin: clinically significant interactions have not been fully elucidated
- Mitoxantrone: clinically significant interactions have not been fully elucidated
- Idarubicin: clinically significant interactions have not been fully elucidated
- Daunorubicin: clinically significant interactions have not been fully elucidated

What are the class adverse effects of the anthracyclines?

- Cardiotoxicity
  - Cumulative
  - Associated with large bolus doses
  - Acute: EKG changes, arrhythmias

– Chronic: heart failure, cardiomyopathy

– Increased risk with prior cardiovascular disease, concurrent cardiotoxic drugs, prior anthracycline therapy, prior or concurrent chest irradiation, older age, and infants/children

– Decreased incidence with liposomal doxorubicin and continuous infusions over 24 to 96 hours

– Epirubicin, idarubicin, and mitoxantrone have less cardiotoxicity

• Myelosuppression, mucositis, alopecia

– More common with prolonged infusions of conventional and liposomal doxorubicin

• Radiosensitization

• Body fluid discoloration (red; except blue for mitoxantrone)

• Secondary malignancies; commonly associated with MLL gene (11q23) rearrangements, which most often occur with a 2- to 3-year latency

• Extravasation

What are the premedications required?

• Premedications (other than standard antiemetics) are not required

What is the emetogenicity level of the anthracyclines?

• Doxorubicin: moderate (<60 mg/m^2) or high (≥ 60 mg/m^2 or in AC regimen)

• Liposomal doxorubicin: low

• Epirubicin: moderate (≤ 90 mg/m^2) or high (>60 mg/m^2)

• Mitoxantrone: low

• Idarubicin: moderate

• Daunorubicin: moderate

Are the anthracyclines vesicants or irritants?

• Vesicants; however liposomal doxorubicin is an irritant

What is the maximum lifetime dose of each anthracycline?

Maximum Lifetime Doses of Anthracyclines

Equivalent Dosing Estimates		Ranges (Doxorubicin: other anthracycline)	Max Below
Doxorubicin	50 mg/m^2	1:1	450
Daunorubicin	50–60 mg/m^2	1:1–1.2	550
Epirubicin	75 mg/m^2	1:1.5–2	900
Idarubicin	10 mg/m^2	1:0.2–0.33	150
Mitoxantrone	12.5 mg/m^2	1:0.25–0.33	140

5

Antimetabolites

ANTIFOLATES

What are the chemotherapy agents in the antifolate class?

- Methotrexate (Trexall®)
- Pemetrexed (Alimta®)
- Pralatrexate (Folotyn®)

What malignancies are the antifolates FDA approved for?

FDA-Approved Uses of Antifolates

Agent	FDA Approval
Methotrexate	Acute lymphoblastic leukemia (ALL), trophoblastic neoplasms (gestational choriocarcinoma, chorioadenoma destruens, and hydatidiform mole), breast cancer, head and neck cancer, cutaneous T-cell lymphoma (CTCL), lung cancer (squamous cell and small cell), non-Hodgkin's lymphomas (NHLs; advanced), osteosarcoma
Pemetrexed	Mesothelioma, non–small cell lung cancer (NSCLC; locally advanced or metastatic nonsquamous; not indicated for squamous cell NSCLC)
Pralatrexate	Peripheral T-cell lymphoma (PTCL; relapsed or refractory)

Abbreviation: FDA, U.S. Food and Drug Administration.

How do the antifolates work? (See Figure 5.1)

• Antifolates disrupt the synthesis of reduced folates, essential cofactors that act as one-carbon carriers in the synthesis of DNA precursors

• Rapidly dividing cells uptake antifolates via the reduced folate carrier system, the folate receptor system, or through a proton-coupled transporter. Methotrexate relies primarily on the reduced folate carrier system for entry, although pralatrexate and pemetrexed have relatively higher affinity for this transporter compared to methotrexate. Pemetrexed is efficiently transported by all three transport mechanisms

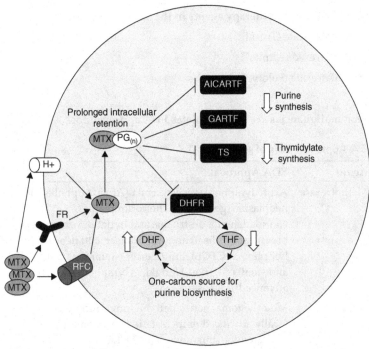

FIGURE 5.1. Antifolates.
Abbreviations: AICARTF, aminoimidazole carboxamide ribonucleotide transformylase; DHF, dihydrofolate; DHFR, dihydrofolate reductase; FR, folate receptor; GARTF, glycinamide ribonucleotide transformylase; H+, proton-coupled transporter; MTX, methotrexate; PG, polyglutamate; RFC, reduced folate carrier; THF, tetrahydrofolate; TS, thymidylate synthase.

- By mimicking the natural folate structure, the antifolate compounds bind and inhibit dihydrofolate reductase (DHFR), a key enzyme in the folate synthesis pathway that normally converts folate into its active, reduced tetrahydrofolate form

- This depletes the pool of reduced folate compounds required for purine analogue synthesis

- Methotrexate and other antifolates are also converted into poly-glutamate derivatives by folylpolyglutamyl synthetase (FPGS). These derivatives are potent inhibitors of other folate-dependent enzymes (eg, aminoimidazole carboxamide ribonucleotide transformylase [AICARTF], glycinamide ribonucleotide transformylase [GARTF], thymidylate synthase [TS]) critical for purine and thymidylate synthesis. Polyglutamated antifolates are also selectively retained within cells, thus prolonging intracellular half-life in tumor cells

- Unlike the other antifolates in clinical use, pemetrexed is a potent inhibitor of TS but a relatively weak inhibitor of DHFR

- Cell cycle phase specific (S-phase)

What are the common mechanisms of resistance to antifolates?

- Decreased transport of antifolates into cancer cells

- Active efflux of antifolates out of cancer cells (eg, multidrug resistance–associated protein [MRP]-1, 2, 3, breast cancer resistance protein [BCRP])

- A reduction in the formation of the polyglutamate forms of the anti-folate compounds

- Mutations in DHFR resulting in reduced antifolate binding affinity

- Increased expression of DHFR within cancer cells

What are the common dosing ranges for the antifolates?

- Methotrexate—Dosing varies widely

  – Orally (PO)/intramuscular (IM)/subcutaneous (SQ): doses vary, 20 mg/m^2 weekly PO for acute lymphoblastic leukemia (ALL)

  – Intrathecal (IT): usually 12 mg (max 15 mg); ½ dose in Ommaya reservoir

– High-dose intravenous (IV) (ALL, diffuse large B-cell lymphoma [DLBCL]): 1 to 3 g/m^2 IV with leucovorin rescue

– Capizzi methotrexate (ALL): Start at 100 mg/m^2 IV, escalate by 50 mg/m^2/dose

– Central nervous system (CNS) lymphoma: 3.5 to 8 g/m^2 IV with leucovorin rescue

– Osteosarcoma: 8 to 14 g/m^2/dose IV with leucovorin rescue

– Breast cancer (CMF): 40 mg/m^2 days 1 and 8 every 4 weeks

• Pemetrexed—500 mg/m^2 IV q21 days

• Pralatrexate—15 to 30 mg/m^2 IV once weekly for 6 weeks of 7-week cycle

Are the antifolates metabolized/eliminated renally or hepatically?

• All of the antifolates are primarily eliminated renally; dose adjust for renal dysfunction

Are there drug interactions with any of the antifolates?

• Drugs that prevent active tubular secretion of antifolates (penicillins [ok to use cephalosporins for febrile neutropenia], probenecid, aspirin/ nonsteroidal anti-inflammatory drugs [NSAIDs], proton pump inhibitors) can delay clearance and increase toxicity. These interactions are most significant with methotrexate, in particular in high-dose regimens.

• Sulfonamides (eg, trimethoprim/sulfamethoxazole [TMP/SMX]) and other drugs that displace methotrexate from albumin binding (eg, salicylates, phenytoin, tetracyclines) may increase the free fraction of methotrexate. The trimethoprim component of TMP/SMX also inhibits DHFR, potentially increasing toxicity in combination with antifolates.

• Asparaginase, when given prior to antifolate compounds such as methotrexate, is antagonistic. The asparaginase products on the market (pegaspargase and *Erwinia* asparaginase) also contain significant glutaminase activity. By depleting glutamine, the formation of antifolate-polyglutamates is greatly reduced, decreasing the efficacy of the antifolate compounds. In contrast, administering methotrexate 4 hours prior to asparaginase (as in the MOAD regimen for ALL) may result in synergistic cytotoxicity.

- Leucovorin rescue in higher doses can abrogate the cytotoxic effects of the antifolate compounds on malignant cells; the minimum dose necessary to prevent host toxicity should be utilized (methotrexate elimination curves to guide leucovorin dosing have been published and are useful in this regard).

- Drugs that inhibit P-glycoprotein (P-gp) may increase methotrexate levels.

- Drugs that decrease renal clearance may increase levels of the antifolates (eg, NSAIDs, calcineurin inhibitors, other nephrotoxic agents).

What are the most common adverse effects of each antifolate?

- Methotrexate (side effects depend on dose and regimen—see table in the following text): myelosuppression, mucositis (usually precedes fall in blood counts), acute kidney injury (renal tubular precipitation and potentially direct renal tubule toxicity), hepatotoxicity (rapid and reversible LFT elevations after high-dose methotrexate; chronic oral therapy may lead to cirrhosis—less common with "pulse" dosing), alopecia, pneumonitis, and three distinct types of neurotoxicity ([a] chemical arachnoiditis—immediate, characterized by headache, nuchal rigidity, vomiting, fever; [b] subacute—typically after three to four courses of IT methotrexate, can lead to motor paralysis, seizures, coma; [c] chronic demyelinating—occurs primarily in children after IT administration, leading to dementia and limb spasticity)

Frequency of Side Effects of Antifolates

Dose in mg/m^2	Heme	Renal	Liver	Mucositis	Lung	Neuro
Intermediate IV continuous infusion 500–1,000	+++	++	++	++	±	−
High-dose IV bolus 3,500–12,000	+	++	++	+	±	++
Low-dose PO daily 5–25	−	−	+++	−	±	−
Low-dose PO pulse	−	−	++	−	±	−
Intrathecal	−	−	−	−	−	++

Note: +++ = very common; − = rare.
Abbreviations: IV, intravenous; PO, orally.

• Pemetrexed: fatigue, myelosuppression, mucositis, rash (can manage/prevent with corticosteroids), increased LFTs, conjunctivitis and increased lacrimation (with long-term use/maintenance therapy)

• Pralatrexate: myelosuppression, nausea/vomiting, mucositis, increased LFTs

What are the premedications and supportive care precautions required?

• High-dose methotrexate (>1 g/m^2): Hydration and urine alkalinization to achieve and maintain urine output of at least 100 mL/hr and a urine pH of 7.0 or greater prior to beginning infusion.

– Methotrexate penetrates into third-space fluid collections, creating a reservoir of methotrexate that prolongs drug half-life leading to significant toxicity. Ensure no fluid collections (eg, ascites, pleural effusions) present prior to and during infusion

– Daily methotrexate drug level monitoring

– Leucovorin rescue beginning 24 to 36 hours after methotrexate infusion initiation (use elimination curves to guide appropriate dosing) until methotrexate levels fall below 0.05 to 0.1 mcg/mL

– In case of delayed elimination and acute kidney injury or other severe toxicity:

○ Increase leucovorin dosing per published elimination curves or institutional guidelines

○ Continue aggressive hydration and urinary alkalinization

○ Consider high-flux hemodialysis to remove methotrexate

○ Consider administering glucarpidase 50 units/kg IV: Glucarpidase is a recombinant bacterial carboxypeptidase that metabolizes methotrexate to the inactive 4-diamino-N(10)-methylpteroic acid (DAMPA) metabolite. The DAMPA metabolite can be detected on methotrexate immunoassay, resulting in falsely high levels of methotrexate; consider high-performance liquid chromatography (HPLC) monitoring in this case. Hold leucovorin 2 to 4 hours before and 1 to 2 hours after glucarpidase, as it can compete with methotrexate for binding to the enzyme. Although glucarpidase is successful in rapidly cleaving methotrexate, the average time to normalization of renal function is still approximately 3 weeks. Aggressive leucovorin rescue remains the most important intervention for delayed methotrexate elimination

• Pemetrexed and pralatrexate: B12 and folic acid supplementation should be provided prior to starting therapy as well as throughout therapy to prevent excessive toxicity.

• Pemetrexed: Dexamethasone 4 mg BID × 3 days starting the day prior to infusion to reduce the incidence of rash.

What is the emetogenicity level of the antifolates?

• The antifolates have a low emetogenic potential

Are the antifolates vesicants or irritants?

• The antifolate compounds are neither vesicants nor irritants

PURINE ANTAGONISTS

What are the chemotherapy agents in the purine antagonist class?
- Mercaptopurine (Purinethol®, 6-MP)
- Thioguanine (Tabloid®)

What malignancies are each purine antagonist FDA approved for?

FDA-Approved Uses of Purine Antagonists

Agent	FDA Approval
Mercaptopurine	Acute lymphoblastic leukemia (ALL)
Thioguanine	Acute myeloid leukemia (however, used more often in ALL)

Abbreviation: FDA, U.S. Food and Drug Administration.

How do the purine antagonists work? (See Figure 5.2)
- Mercaptopurine and thioguanine are metabolized through independent pathways to thioguanine monophosphate (TGMP), which is then metabolized in several steps to active thioguanine nucleotides (6-deoxy-thioguanosine triphosphate)
  - Incorporated into DNA or RNA, interfere with DNA/RNA replication, and induce cytotoxicity
- Also inhibit de novo purine synthesis (by methylmercaptopurine nucleotides)
  - Less inhibition from 6-TG than 6-MP
- The primary enzyme involved in their activation is hypoxanthine-guanine phosphoribosyltransferase (HGPRT)
- The primary enzyme involved in their deactivation is thiopurine methyltransferase (TPMT)
  - See TPMT deficiency clinical pearls at end of chapter
- Cell cycle specific (S phase)

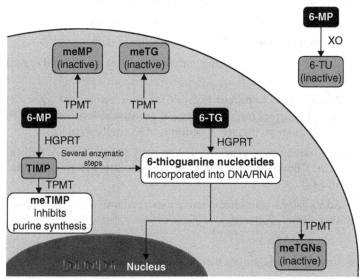

FIGURE 5.2. Purine antagonists: Intracellularly, 6-mercaptopurine (6-MP) and 6-thioguanine (6-TG) are processed by both a catabolic and an anabolic pathway. Catabolically, both are methylated and inactivated by thiopurine methyltransferase (TPMT) to methyl-MP (meMP) and methyl-TG (meTG). Hypoxanthine-guanine phosphoribosyltransferase (HGPRT) converts 6-MP to thioinosine monophosphate (TIMP). TIMP is further converted to methyl-TIMP (meTIMP) via TPMT and has the ability to inhibit purine synthesis. TIMP is also converted via several enzymatic steps to active metabolites, 6-thioguanine nucleotides. These are incorporated into DNA/RNA and ultimately lead to apoptosis. 6-TG is directly converted to 6-thioguanine nucleotides. 6-thioguanine nucleotides also undergo catabolism to be inactivated via TPMT. 6-MP is also converted to an inactive metabolite, 6-thiouric acid (6-TU), via xanthine oxidase (XO).

What are the common mechanisms of resistance to purine antagonists?

• The most extensively characterized mechanism of resistance is the reduced activity of HGPRT

• Reduced influx by transporter cells

• Increased expression of TPMT (although decreased expression is more common)

What are the common dosing ranges for each purine antagonist?

- Mercaptopurine: Various treatment regimens exist:

  - Maintenance for ALL: 50 mg PO three times daily

  - 60 to 80 mg/m²/day during various courses of ALL (round to nearest 25 mg)

  - Absorption is improved if given 1/2 hour before or 1 hour after meals. Concurrent milk products can decrease absorption and 6-MP effect is enhanced if given at bedtime on an empty stomach

- Thioguanine: 60 mg/m²/day PO on days 29 to 42 for CALGB10403 and CALGB8811 (Larson protocol) during delayed intensification (Course IV)

  - Administer 1 hour after evening meal, preferably at bedtime (avoid milk or citrus products)

Are the purine antagonists metabolized/eliminated renally or hepatically?

- Both are extensively metabolized hepatically via first pass; however, a high interpatient variability exists; therefore, no formal dosing recommendations for patients with liver dysfunction; in severe dysfunction, it is generally held until resolution since mercaptopurine/thioguanine can exacerbate hepatic impairment

  - 6-MP is metabolized via methylation (via TPMT) and oxidation in the liver (also metabolized by xanthine oxidase)

  - 6-TG is metabolized via deamination and methylation (via TPMT) in the liver (it is NOT metabolized by xanthine oxidase)

- Both are renally excreted; however, no formal dose reduction exists for patients with renal impairment

Are there drug interactions with any of the purine antagonists?

- Mercaptopurine: Allopurinol inhibits xanthine oxidase and therefore inhibits metabolism of mercaptopurine (avoid use or reduce initial mercaptopurine by 33% in ALL regimens and dose adjust for response and toxicity)

• Mercaptopurine: Warfarin's anticoagulant effects may be decreased; unknown mechanism; monitor international normalized ratio (INR) and adjust warfarin

• Mercaptopurine and thioguanine: Mesalamine, sulfasalazine, olsalazine can inhibit TPMT

What are the most common adverse effects of each purine antagonist?

• Mercaptopurine: • myelosuppression (primarily leukopenia and thrombocytopenia); gastrointestinal toxicities (stomatitis, diarrhea, abdominal pain); and hepatotoxicity

• Thioguanine: myelosuppression (more than 6-MP); gastrointestinal toxicities are less than 6-MP (stomatitis, diarrhea, abdominal pain); splenomegaly; and hepatotoxicity

What is the emetogenicity level of the purine antagonists?

• Both agents have minimal to low emetogenicity

What is TPMT deficiency and what are some clinical pearls regarding it?

• Diminished TPMT activity leads to a shunting of TGMP metabolism toward greater production of active thioguanine nucleotides

• When treated with full-dose therapy, 35% of TPMT heterozygous patients and 100% of homozygous patients will require dose reductions, compared with only 7% of patients without mutations

• One in 300 patients has complete TPMT deficiency, and 11% carry a single defective allele

• TPMT deficiency is diagnosed according to either phenotypic testing of erythrocyte TPMT activity and/or genotyping for TPMT gene mutations

• Use of preemptive genotyping is recommended; however, in those with unknown TPMT activity who experience disproportionate myelosuppression (>2 weeks), genotyping should be conducted

• Patients identified as TPMT deficient receive either empiric dose reduction or full-dose therapy with enhanced myelotoxicity monitoring

Recommended Starting Dosing of Mercaptopurine and Thioguanine in Patients With TPMT Variants

TPMT Genotype	Mercaptopurine Dosing	Thioguanine Dosing
Heterozygous	30%–70% of full dose 2–4 weeks to reach steady state	50%–70% of full dose 2–4 weeks to reach steady state
Homozygous	10% of full dose given three times/week 4–6 weeks to reach steady state	10% of full dose given three times/week 4–6 weeks to reach steady state

Abbreviation: TPMT, thiopurine methyltransferase.

Source: Adapted from Relling MV, Gardner EE, Sandborn WJ, et al. Clinical pharmacogenetics implementation consortium guidelines for thiopurine methyltransferase genotype and thiopurine dosing: 2013 update. *Clin Pharmacol Ther*. 2013;93:324–325. Copyright John Wiley and Sons, used with permission.

PURINE ANALOGUES

What are the chemotherapy agents in the purine analogue class?

- Cladribine (Leustatin®)
- Clofarabine (Clolar®)
- Fludarabine (Fludara®)
- Nelarabine (Arranon®)
- Pentostatin (Nipent®)

What malignancies are each purine analogue FDA approved for?

FDA-Approved Uses of Purine Analogues

Agent	FDA Approval
Cladribine	Hairy cell leukemia
Clofarabine	Pediatric acute lymphoblastic leukemia (ALL) (ages 1 to 21 y); relapsed refractory ALL
Fludarabine	Chronic lymphocytic leukemia
Nelarabine	Relapsed/refractory T-cell ALL and T-cell lymphoblastic lymphoma
Pentostatin	Hairy cell leukemia

Abbreviation: FDA, U.S. Food and Drug Administration.

How do the purine analogues work?

- Cladribine, clofarabine, and fludarabine mimic deoxyadenosine, while nelarabine mimics deoxyguanosine

- All are activated inside the cell to 5′-triphosphate form, incorporated into DNA, and inhibit chain elongation by inhibiting DNA polymerase

- Their structure (chloride and/or fluoride additions) makes them resistant to their respective deaminases

- The purine analogues also inhibit ribonucleotide reductase activity, decreasing the production of normal deoxyribonucleotides (dNTPs) available for DNA synthesis

- Due to a reduction in the dNTP pools, inhibition of ribonucleotide reductase also enhances deoxycytidine kinase, which is the rate-limiting enzyme in purine/pyrimidine phosphorylation into DNA

  – This is the premise behind administering a purine analogue 4 hours prior to cytarabine

  – Higher deoxycytidine kinase leads to higher active triphosphate metabolite of cytarabine (arabinofuranosylcytosine triphosphate [ara-CTP]) = synergy

- Clofarabine can also directly affect the mitochondrion altering the transmembrane potential and releasing cytochrome C, which leads to apoptosis via the apoptosome

- Pentostatin is an adenosine deaminase inhibitor, leading to the accumulation of cytotoxic deoxyadenosine triphosphate, which inhibits ribonucleotide reductase, as well as DNA methylation, replication, and repair, ultimately resulting in apoptosis

What are the common mechanisms of resistance to purine analogue therapy?

- Decreased drug transport into cells
- Decreased expression of deoxycytidine kinase
- Increased expression of ribonucleotide reductase

What are the common dosing ranges for purine analogues?

Cladribine:

- Hairy cell: 0.09 mg/kg/day IV × 7 days (continuous infusion), repeat every 28 to 35 days
- Chronic lymphocytic leukemia (CLL): 0.1 mg/kg/day × 7 days OR 0.028 to 0.14 mg/kg/day × 5 days
- Chronic myeloid leukemia (CML): 15 mg/m²/day × 5 days
- Acute myeloid leukemia (AML): 5 mg/m²/day × 5 days

Clofarabine:

- Acute lymphoblastic leukemia (ALL): 52 mg/m² IV over 2 hours daily × 5 days every 2 to 6 weeks

- AML: 15 to 40 mg/m^2 IV daily × 5 days every 4 to 6 weeks (monotherapy)
- Bone marrow transplant (BMT): 40 mg/m^2

Fludarabine:

- 25 mg/m^2 IV × 5 days every 28 days

Nelarabine:

- 1,500 mg/m^2/day over 2 hours on days 1, 3, and 5; repeat every 21 days; pediatric dosing is 650 mg/m^2/day over 1 hour on days 1 to 5

Pentostatin:

- Hairy cell: 4 mg/m^2 every 2 weeks
- CLL: 2 mg/m^2 (first line) or 4 mg/m^2 (salvage) weekly every 3 weeks × 6 weeks
- T-cell lymphoma: 3.75 to 5 mg/m^2 daily for 3 days every 3 weeks
- Graft-versus-host disease (GVHD): 1.5 mg/m^2 daily for 3 days (acute); 4 mg/m^2 every 2 weeks × 12 doses (chronic)

Are the purine analogues metabolized/eliminated renally or hepatically?

- All purine analogues are renally eliminated

Are there drug interactions with any of the purine analogues?

- Cladribine: ethanol—gastrointestinal (GI) irritation
- Clofarabine: azole antifungals—increased hepatotoxicity
- Fludarabine: cytarabine (increased activity); cyclophosphamide, cisplatin, mitoxantrone (increased activity); pentostatin—increases drug levels and pulmonary toxicity
- Nelarabine: pentostatin—decreases drug levels
- Pentostatin: fludarabine—pulmonary toxicity; nelarabine—reduced efficacy; cyclophosphamide—increased risk of cardiac toxicity

What is the purine analogue class adverse effect?

- Myelosuppression

What are the adverse effects of each purine analogue?

- Cladribine: myelosuppression with longer duration of nadir (recover 4 to 8 weeks), fever, rash; neurotoxicity with high doses of continuous infusion

- Clofarabine: hepatotoxicity (usually within days and reversible in 14 days), rash, capillary leak syndrome

- Fludarabine: autoimmune hemolytic anemia/thrombocytopenia, idiopathic thrombocytopenic purpura

- Nelarabine: central nervous system (dose-limiting toxicity; headache, altered mental status, seizures, somnolence, convulsions, peripheral neuropathy), peripheral edema, hepatotoxicity

- Pentostatin: neurotoxicity (doses >4 mg/m^2) (headache, lethargy, fatigue), nephrotoxicity, fever, fatigue, rash, myalgia; hepatotoxicity

Which are the premedications required?

- No routine premedications (other than standard antiemetics) required

What is the emetogenicity level of the purine analogues?

- Clofarabine is moderate
- Cladribine, fludarabine, and nelarabine are minimal
- Pentostatin is low

Are the purine analogues vesicants or irritants?

- Cladribine is an irritant
- All others are nonvesicants/nonirritants

PYRIMIDINE ANALOGUES/FLUOROPYRIMIDINES

What are the chemotherapy agents in this class?

- Fluorouracil (5-FU) (Adrucil®)
- Capecitabine (Xeloda®)—prodrug of 5-FU
- Floxuridine (FUDR®)

What malignancies are each fluoropyrimidine analogue FDA approved for?

FDA-Approved Uses of Fluoropyrimidine Analogues

Agent	FDA Approval
Fluorouracil (5-FU)	Carcinoma of the breast, pancreas, colon, rectum, and stomach
Capecitabine	Adjuvant colon cancer, metastatic colorectal cancer, and metastatic breast cancer
Floxuridine	Gastric and colorectal cancer metastatic to the liver

Abbreviation: FDA, U.S. Food and Drug Administration.

How do fluoropyrimidine analogues work? (Figure 5.3)

- Interfere with DNA synthesis, RNA synthesis, and/or thymidylate synthetase (TS) resulting in apoptosis

How does the metabolism/mechanisms of each agent differ?

- 5-fluorouracil is converted to three main metabolites (5-fluorouridine triphosphate [5-FUTP], which is incorporated into RNA, 5-fluoro-deoxyuridine triphosphate [5-FdUTP], which is incorporated into DNA, and 5-fluorodeoxyuridine monophosphate [5-FdUMP], which inhibits thymidylate synthetase)

  – Of note, leucovorin is metabolized to 5-methyl-tetrahydrofolate, which stabilizes the bond between FdUMP and TS. This enhances TS inhibition and decreases the production of thymidylate

- Capecitabine is enzymatically converted in the liver and tissues to 5-FU

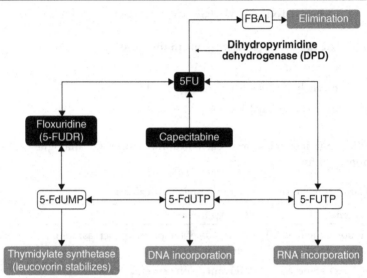

FIGURE 5.3. Pyrimidine analogues: Capecitabine (cape) is an oral prodrug metabolized to fluorouracil (5-FU). 5-FU is intracellularly bioactivated (anabolic pathway) through several steps to 5-fluorodeoxyuridine monophosphate (5-FdUMP), which inhibits thymidylate synthetase (TS), causing cellular cytotoxicity. Leucovorin metabolizes to 5-methyl-tetrahydrofolate, which stabilizes the bond between FdUMP and TS. This enhances TS inhibition and decreases the production of thymidylate. Fluorodeoxyuridine triphosphate (5-FdUTP) and fluorouridine triphosphate (5-FUTP) are incorporated into DNA and RNA, respectively, as false base pairs. Floxuridine (5-FUDR) is a metabolite of 5-FU and a precursor to 5-FdUMP, which ultimately inhibits TS or can be converted back into 5-FU. The rate-limiting step for 5-FU elimination is an alternative metabolic pathway (catabolic pathway) catalyzed by dihydropyrimidine dehydrogenase (DPD). Majority of 5-FU will follow the catabolic pathway; therefore, deficiencies in DPD can lead to severe toxicities as more active metabolites will be created.

- Floxuridine (5-FUDR) is converted to FdUTP (incorporated into DNA) and FdUMP (inhibits TS)
  - Rationale for use in liver metastases:
    ○ When liver metastases grow above 2 to 3 mm, the blood supply is delivered from the hepatic artery (not portal circulation)

○ Drugs that are highly extracted by the liver during first-pass metabolism can result in high hepatic levels and low systemic concentrations, thereby minimizing systemic toxicity

○ The best drugs for hepatic arterial infusion (HAI) are agents that have high hepatic extraction with conversion to inactive metabolites, high total body clearance, and short plasma half-life

○ If the drug is not rapidly cleared by the liver, the regional advantage is lost because of systemic recirculation

What are common mechanisms of resistance to fluoropyrimidine analogue therapy?

• Increased production of TS, p53 mutations, efflux pumps, increase in uridine production, decreased levels of reduced folate cofactor, DNA repair mechanisms, decreased incorporation of 5-FU into RNA/DNA, dihydropyrimidine dehydrogenase (DPD) overexpression

What are the common dosing ranges for each fluoropyrimidine analogue?

• 5-FU: Bolus (200 to 800 mg/m^2); continuous infusion (200 to 2,600 mg/m^2/day); radiosensitization (300 mg/m^2/day)

– Clinical pearl: Leucovorin helps stabilize 5-FU binding and inhibition of TS with bolus dosing due to the short half-life of 5-FU, but there is no evidence it is necessary with continuous infusion of 5-FU or with capecitabine

• Capecitabine: 850 to 1,250 mg/m^2 BID × 2 weeks, then 1 week of rest. Taken orally 30 minutes after a meal; radiosensitization (1,650 mg/m^2/day split BID on days of radiation)

• Floxuridine: 0.1 to 0.6 mg/kg/day or 4 to 20 mg/day intra-arterial × 7 to 14 days

Are the pyrimidine analogues metabolized/eliminated renally or hepatically?

• Hepatic metabolism via a dehydrogenase enzyme

– Metabolism is not via cytochrome p450 enzymes or glucuronidation

– No FDA-approved labeling dose adjustments

- Renally adjust for capecitabine (contraindicated if creatinine clearance <30 mL/min)

Are there drug interactions with any of the fluoropyrimidine analogues?

- 5-FU: inhibits CYP2C9; leucovorin (enhances antitumor activity/toxicity of bolus, not infusion)
- Capecitabine: inhibits CYP2C9 (eg, warfarin, phenytoin)
- Floxuridine: leucovorin (enhances antitumor activity/toxicity)

What are the most common adverse effects of each fluoropyrimidine analogue?

IV Bolus 5-FU	Continuous Infusion 5-FU/Capecitabine
Myelosuppression (dose-limiting toxicity [DLT])	Less myelosuppression
Mucositis (higher incidence)	*Mucositis (more severe)*
Diarrhea (more severe)	*Diarrhea (higher incidence)*
Hand-foot syndrome is uncommon	*Hand-foot syndrome*

Note: Other notable toxicities: fingernail discoloration, discoloration from IV infusion (veins turn gray), conjunctivitis, hair loss or thinning, phototoxicity, cardiotoxicity (coronary vasospasm, angina, dysrhythmias, cardiogenic shock, sudden death, ECG changes, and cardiomyopathy), neurotoxicity (mood changes, depression, confusion, hallucinations, nervousness, difficulty sleeping, dizziness, drowsiness, clumsiness, difficulty walking, or restlessness).

Abbreviations: 5-FU, fluorouracil; IV, intravenous.

FLOXURIDINE

Local and regional effects of intra-arterial infusion

- Floxuridine is metabolized to fluorouracil, but the full spectrum of fluorouracil toxicity is not expected due to regional administration of the drug

- Arterial aneurysm, arterial ischemia, arterial thrombosis, bleeding at catheter site, blocked/displaced/leaking catheter, embolism, fibromyositis, infection at catheter site, hepatic necrosis, abscesses, and thrombophlebitis

- Peptic ulcer disease, gastritis, biliary sclerosis, chemical hepatitis, cholecystitis

What are the premedications required?

- Premedication is not required for any of the agents

What is the emetogenicity level of the fluoropyrimidine analogues?

- All are classified as low emetogenic risk

Are fluoropyrimidine analogues vesicants or irritants?

- 5-FU is an irritant

Clinical Pearl: What is DPD deficiency and how does it affect fluoropyrimidine therapy?

- Normally, most of 5-FU/capecitabine is not bioactivated and instead converted to inactive metabolites by DPD and eliminated

- Patients with lower DPD activity have a higher propensity for life-threatening toxicities (myelosuppression, gastrointestinal toxicity, mucositis/stomatitis, and hand-foot syndrome)

PYRIMIDINE ANALOGUES/DEOXYCYTIDINE ANALOGUES

What are the chemotherapy agents in this class?

- Deoxycytidine analogues
  - Cytarabine
  - Gemcitabine (Gemzar®)

What malignancies are each deoxycytidine analogue FDA approved for?

FDA-Approved Uses of Deoxycytidine Analogues

Agent	Approval
Cytarabine	Acute myeloid leukemia (AML), acute lymphoblastic leukemia (ALL), chronic myeloid leukemia (CML) (blast phase), meningeal leukemia
Gemcitabine	Non–small cell lung cancer (NSCLC), pancreatic, metastatic breast, ovarian cancer

Abbreviation: FDA, U.S. Food and Drug Administration.

How do deoxycytidine analogues work?

- Cytarabine is activated to the nucleotide metabolite arabinofuranosylcytosine triphosphate (ara-CTP) by deoxycytidine kinase and incorporated into DNA
  - Also inhibits DNA polymerase α and weakly inhibits ribonucleotide reductase (see Figure 5.4)
  - Cell cycle specific to the S Phase
- Gemcitabine is activated intracellularly by deoxycytidine kinase and is incorporated into DNA as a false base pair
  - Also inhibits ribonucleotide reductase, which leads to decreased production of dNTPs and increased deoxycytidine kinase activity
  - Cell cycle specific to the S phase

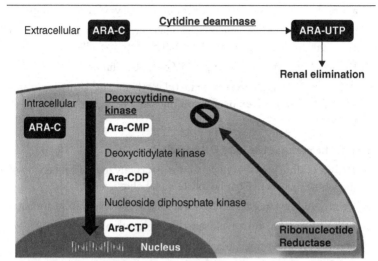

FIGURE 5.4. Cytarabine MOA and metabolism: Extracellular cytarabine (ara-C) is transported via an active transport system (human equilibrative nucleoside transporter 1 [hENT1]) when given in a low dose (100–200 mg/m^2) continuous infusion and by passive diffusion when given at high doses (1,000–3,000 mg/m^2). ara-C must be converted to its active metabolite ara-CTP. The rate-limiting step in the activation of ara-C is via deoxycytidine kinase. ara-CTP is incorporated into DNA during S phase of the cell cycle. Extracellularly, ara-C is degraded by cytidine deaminase (present in granulocytes, leukemia cells, plasma, liver, spleen, and red blood cells) into ara-UTP and renally eliminated. Patients with poor renal function can accumulate ara-UTP and exhibit symptoms of cerebellar neurotoxicity.
Abbreviation: MOA, Mechanism of Action.

What are the common mechanisms of resistance to deoxycytidine analogue therapy?

• Cytarabine: increased cytidine deaminase, increased deoxycytidylate deaminase, decreased transport into the cell (reduced expression of the human equilibrative nucleoside transporter 1, increased expression of CTP synthetase)

• Gemcitabine: similar to cytarabine

What are the common dose ranges for each deoxycytidine analogue?

- Cytarabine: 100 to 200 mg/m^2/day via continuous IV infusion; high dose—1,000 to 3,000 mg/m^2 IV; 25 to 100 mg intrathecally
- Gemcitabine: 800 to 1,200 mg/m^2 IV over 30 minutes
  - May be given as a fixed dose rate (FDR) (10 mg/m^2/min); for example, 900 mg/m^2 is given over 90 minutes or 700 mg/m^2 is given over 70 minutes

What is the premise behind FDR gemcitabine?

- Deoxycytidine kinase is the enzyme that catalyzes the conversion of gemcitabine to its active triphosphate metabolite
- Deoxycytidine kinase is saturated at the standard 30-minute infusion
- FDR of 10 mg/m^2/min avoids enzyme saturation
- Permits greater intracellular accumulation

Are the deoxycytidine analogues metabolized/eliminated renally or hepatically?

- Metabolism is not via cytochrome p450 enzymes or glucuronidation
- Renally adjust for high-dose cytarabine (not required for 100–200 mg/m^2 continuous infusion dosing)
  - Extracellularly, cytarabine is converted to ara-U (neurotoxic metabolite) via cytidine deaminase
    - ara-U is eliminated renally

Are there drug interactions with any of the deoxycytidine analogues?

- Cytarabine:
  - Purine analogues (fludarabine, clofarabine, cladribine) enhance deoxycitidine kinase and inhibit riboucleotide reductase, thus increasing conversion of cytarabine to active ara-CTP
  - 5-FU—cytarabine reduces efficacy of 5-FU
  - Methotrexate—increases ara-CTP formation/activity of cytarabine
  - Alkylating agents—alkylators inhibit DNA repair, increasing cytarabine cytotoxicity
- Gemcitabine: cisplatin (enhances cytotoxicity of cisplatin), also a potent radiosensitizer

What are the most common adverse effects of each deoxycytidine analogue?

- Gemcitabine: myelosuppression (all three lineages), flulike symptoms and fever, peripheral edema, LFT abnormalities, dyspnea and pulmonary toxicity, infusion reactions, transient rash (typically erythematous, pruritic, and maculopapular; reversible and respond to local therapy)

- Cytarabine:

Standard-Dose ara-C	High-Dose ara-C (1–3 g/m^2)
Myelosuppression	Myelosuppression
Nausea—low	Nausea—moderate
Diarrhea	More diarrhea
Mucositis	Mucositis
Alopecia	*Neurotoxicity (cerebellar)*
	Rash
	Conjunctivitis (requires steroid eye drops)
	Alopecia

- Other ara-C side effects: hand-foot syndrome, hepatotoxicity, ara-C syndrome (fever, myalgia, bone pain, maculopapular rash, malaise)

What are the clinical features of cytarabine-induced cerebellar toxicity?

- **Symptoms:** gait ataxia, nystagmus, dysmetria, dysarthria (slurred speech), and somnolence; rarely: seizure, coma, cerebral dysfunction

- **Risk factors:** age, cumulative dose, renal and hepatic dysfunction, rate of administration, CNS involvement, previous neurotoxicity from ara-C

- **Time period:** usually occurs between the 3rd and 8th day of therapy and typically resolves in 3 to 10 days (sometimes can persist and be fatal)

- **Prevention/treatment:** hemodialysis to remove neurotoxic ara-U metabolite

What are the premedications required?

- Premedication is not required for any of the agents

What is the emetogenicity level of the deoxycytidine analogues?

- Moderate risk: cytarabine (>200 mg/m^2)
- Low risk: gemcitabine, cytarabine (≤200 mg/m^2)

Are deoxycytidine analogues vesicants or irritants?

- Gemcitabine is an irritant

II

Next-Generation Antineoplastics

Monoclonal Antibodies

What is a monoclonal antibody?

- Protein (immunoglobulin) produced by memory B cells (or plasma cells) that binds to a specific epitope

- As a *monoclonal* antibody (as opposed to *polyclonal* antibody), it has monovalent affinity—meaning it binds to one specific epitope

What are the various isotypes of antibodies?

- Immunoglobulin G (IgG; IgG1 through 4), IgA (IgA 1 through 2), IgM, IgD, IgE

- Therapeutic monoclonal antibodies are of the IgG isotype

How do monoclonal antibodies induce cytotoxicity in target cells? (Refer to Figure 8.1)

- Antibody-dependent cell-mediated cytotoxicity (ADCC): An effector cell (eg, natural killer [NK] cells, monocytes, macrophages) recognizes the antibody bound to the target cell through Fc receptors and destroys the target cell.

- Complement-dependent cytotoxicity (CDC): Antibody bound to the target cell activates the complement cascade via the classical pathway, ultimately leading to the formation of the membrane attack complex and lysis of the cell.

- Direct killing: Binding of antibody to the epitope on target cells leads to transmission of intracellular signals resulting in apoptosis or programmed cell death.

How are monoclonal antibodies named?

Flowchart of How Monoclonal Antibodies Are Named

1. Prefix unique to drug				
2. Target/ disease class	-tu-, -t- = tumor	-li-, -l- = immunomodulator	-ki-, -k- = interleukins	-ne-, -n- = neurons as target
	-so-, -s- = bone	-ci-, -c- = circulatory system	-vi-, -v- = antiviral	-ba-, -b- = bacterial
	-gro-, -gr- = growth factor	-tox-, -toxa- = toxin	-fu-, -f- = fungus	
3. Antibody source	-o- = mouse (100% foreign)	-xi- = chimeric (~75% human/~25% foreign)	-zu- = humanized (~95% human/~5% foreign)	-u- = human = fully human (100% human)
4. Suffix = mab				

Are there drug interactions with any of the monoclonal antibodies?

• Monoclonal antibodies are not metabolized via cytochrome P450; therefore no classic, pharmacokinetic drug interactions exist

• Pharmacodynamic interactions are dependent on the specific monoclonal antibody and its pharmacologic effects

Are the monoclonal antibodies metabolized/eliminated renally or hepatically?

• No renal or hepatic metabolism/elimination; therefore no dose adjustments necessary

• Typically eliminated by the reticuloendothelial system

Are the monoclonal antibodies vesicants or irritants?

- Ado-trastuzumab emtansine is classified as an irritant, as reactions secondary to extravasation have occurred

- Other monoclonal antibodies are classified as nonvesicants and non-irritants

What is the emetogenicity level of the monoclonal antibodies?

- Low emetogenicity

What are the agents in the monoclonal antibody class?

Agents in the Monoclonal Antibody Class

Name	FDA-Approved Indication	Target	Dose Range	Toxicities (notable)	Comments
Alemtuzumab (Campath®)	CLL, relapsed multiple sclerosis (Lemtrada®)	CD52	CLL: 30 mg IV/ subcutaneous TIW × 4–12 weeks (titrate up on first cycle; 3 mg, 10 mg, 30 mg)	• Pancytopenia • Infusion reactions and fever • Headache, fatigue, skin rash, infections (monitor CMV/EBV) • Autoimmune thyroid disease • Antibody development (not associated with decreased efficacy) • Increase in malignancy (thyroid cancer, melanoma, and lymphoma)	• Prophylaxis: herpes simplex and *Pneumocystis jirovecii* • Premedicate: acetaminophen + Benadryl ± glucocorticoids • Not commercially available—Campath Distribution Program • Reinitiate dose escalation if treatment withheld for ≥7 days • Available as subcutaneous route for CLL, which may have more injection site reactions and may require a longer dose escalation

(continued)

Agents in the Monoclonal Antibody Class (*continued*)

Name	FDA-Approved Indication	Target	Dose Range	Toxicities (notable)	Comments
Bevacizumab (Avastin®)	Cervical cancer, colorectal cancer, glioblastoma, nonsquamous NSCLC, ovarian cancer, fallopian tube cancer, primary peritoneal cancer, renal cell carcinoma	VEGF	5-15 mg/kg IV q2-3 weeks	• Black box warning: hemorrhage, GI perforation, compromised wound healing • Fistula formation, wound dehiscence, peripheral edema, venous and arterial thrombotic effects, proteinuria	• Hold around surgery • Potentiates concomitant chemotherapy toxicities
Blinatumomab (Blincyto™) [bi-specific T-cell engager]	ALL	CD3-CD19	First cycle: 9 mcg/day × 7 days, then 28 mcg/day × 21 days Subsequent cycles: 28 mcg daily × 28 days	• Cytokine release syndrome • Neurotoxicity • B-cell aplasia • Tumor lysis syndrome • Infection, fever	• Premedicate: IV dexamethasone • Hospitalize for first 9 days on cycle 1 • Short half-life; therefore is a continuous infusion pump that needs to be changed every 24-48 hours

(continued)

Agents in the Monoclonal Antibody Class (continued)

Name	FDA-Approved Indication	Target	Dose Range	Toxicities (notable)	Comments
Brentuximab vedotin (Adcetris®) [Antibody-drug conjugate]	Refractory HL, systemic anaplastic large cell lymphoma	CD30	1.8 mg/kg (max 180 mg) q3 weeks	• Black box warning: JC virus • Peripheral neuropathy (sensory and motor), neutropenia, and thrombocytopenia • Hepatotoxicity, tumor lysis syndrome, infusion-related reactions possible, skin rash	• Premeds: acetaminophen, antihistamine • Contraindicated with bleomycin due to pulmonary toxicity • Antibody-drug conjugate: (a) CD30 antibody, (b) MMAE (microtubule inhibitor), (c) protease-cleavable dipeptide linker • Induces cell cycle arrest in G2/M • MMAE is metabolized via CYP3A4 and renally eliminated (no data to suggest dose modifications)

(continued)

Agents in the Monoclonal Antibody Class (continued)

Name	FDA-Approved Indication	Target	Dose Range	Toxicities (notable)	Comments
Cetuximab (Erbitux®)	Metastatic colorectal cancer KRAS WT, head and neck squamous cell	EGFR	400 mg/m^2 LD, then 250 mg/m^2 weekly. If concurrent with radiation, give 1 dose/week (off-label 500 mg/m^2 every 2 weeks)	• Black box warning: infusion reactions, cardiopulmonary arrest • Fatigue, skin rash (acneiform, erythema, pruritus), hand-foot syndrome, diarrhea, periungual/nail alterations, hypomagnesemia, nausea, warning for cardiopulmonary arrest with XRT, interstitial lung disease, trichomegaly and poliosis of the eyelashes	• Premeds: acetaminophen, antihistamine • Anti-cetuximab antibodies form in 5% of patients; unclear if this affects efficacy • High prevalence of hypersensitivity reactions to cetuximab in Southeastern United States (Tennessee, North Carolina, Virginia, Missouri, Arkansas)—due to IgE antibody against galactose-α-1, 3-galactose present on Fab portion of cetuximab (not present in panitumumab)

(continued)

Agents in the Monoclonal Antibody Class (*continued*)

Name	FDA-Approved Indication	Target	Dose Range	Toxicities (notable)	Comments
Denosumab (Xgeva®)	Prevention of skeletal-related events in patients with bone metastasis from solid tumors, giant cell tumor of the bone, osteoporosis/bone loss (Prolia®)	RANKL	120 mg subcutaneous every 4 weeks Osteoporosis/bone loss—60 mg subcutaneous every 6 months	Hypocalcemia, bone fractures, rash, osteonecrosis of the jaw, musculoskeletal pain, fatigue	• Prevents osteoclastic bone resorption • Administer with vitamin D and calcium • Caution in renal impairment
Dinutuximab (Unituxin™)	Neuroblastoma (pediatric)	GD2	17.5 mg/m² / day × 4 days × 5 cycles (on different days of cycle depending on odd or even cycle)	Extreme pain, peripheral neuropathy, bone marrow suppression, capillary leak syndrome, hypotension, hyponatremia, hypokalemia, hypocalcemia, syndrome of inappropriate antidiuretic, ocular toxicity, HUS	• ADCC and CDC • Premeds: opioids, hydration, antihistamine ± acetaminophen • Requires pain management because GD2 is expressed on nerves

(*continued*)

Agents in the Monoclonal Antibody Class (continued)

Name	FDA-Approved Indication	Target	Dose Range	Toxicities (notable)	Comments
Eculizumab (Soliris®)	Atypical HUS, PNH	C5 complement protein	900 mg (600 mg) weekly × 4 doses, then 1,200 mg (900 mg) every 2 weeks ( ) = PNH dosing	• Infections with encapsulated organisms and aspergillus, hypertension, peripheral edema, headache, diarrhea, nausea	• Vaccinate for encapsulated organisms • Blocks formation of C5b thereby inhibiting the formation of the terminal membrane attack complex C5b-9, preventing complement-induced cell death
Gemtuzumab ozogamicin (Mylotarg®) [Antibody-drug conjugate]	(approved for AML but pulled from market) potential future uses APL, AML	CD33	6–9 mg/m² q14–28 days × 2 doses	• Cerebral hemorrhage, bone marrow suppression, hepatotoxicity including veno-occlusive disease, pulmonary toxicity (higher risk with WBC > 30)	• Premeds: acetaminophen, antihistamine • Due to safety concerns and lack of clinical benefit, withdrawn from the market • Antibody-drug conjugate: (a) CD33 antibody, (b) calicheamicin (antitumor antibiotic) • Antibody-drug conjugate delivered into cell upon binding to CD33 via endocytosis • Covalent link is hydrolyzed in the acidic cellular environment and calicheamicin is released. G2/M cell cycle arrest

(continued)

Agents in the Monoclonal Antibody Class (*continued*)

Name	FDA-Approved Indication	Target	Dose Range	Toxicities (notable)	Comments
Ibritumomab tiuxetan (Zevalin®) [Antibody-radioisotope conjugate]	Relapsed/refractory, low-grade or follicular NHL, previously untreated follicular NHL patients who achieve a partial or complete response to first-line chemotherapy	CD20	Within 4 hours of rituximab -Plts >150,000: 0.4 mCi/kg -Plts <100,000–150,000: 0.3 mCi/kg (max 32 mCi)	• Black box warning: bone marrow suppression, thrombocytopenia (nadir 50 days), neutropenia (nadir 60 days), anemia (nadir 70 days), infusion reactions, and mucocutaneous reactions • Secondary malignancies and MDS, respiratory reactions, radiation necrosis, delayed radiation injury (1 month)	• B-cell recovery in 3 months • Antibody-drug conjugate: (a) CD20 antibody, (b) tiuxetan chelator that binds the yttrium-90 (radioactive isotope)—β-emission induces in vitro apoptosis due to free radical formation in CD20 cells and in lymphoid cells/nodules/organs • Affects surrounding cells due to path length of 100–200 cells (collateral damage) • Avoid in plts <100
Ipilimumab (Yervoy®)	Unresectable metastatic melanoma	CTLA-4	3 mg/kg IV q3 weeks × 4 doses	• Black box warning: induces GVHD-like symptoms (enterocolitis, hepatitis, dermatitis, endocrinopathies)	• CTLA-4 downregulates T-cell activation; blockade of CTLA-4 allows T-cell activation and proliferation • Clinical response and toxicities take weeks to months to manifest

(*continued*)

Agents in the Monoclonal Antibody Class (*continued*)

Name	FDA-Approved Indication	Target	Dose Range	Toxicities (notable)	Comments
				• Fatigue, headache, nausea, diarrhea, rare but fatal neurotoxicity (hypophysitis)	• Manage severe (grade 3–4) toxicities with high-dose corticosteroids; may require other immunosuppressants if refractory (eg, TNF-α inhibitors, mycophenolic acid)
Nivolumab (Opdivo®)	Unresectable or metastatic melanoma with progression following ipilimumab and a BRAF inhibitor, metastatic squamous cell NSCLC progressed on platinum chemotherapy	PD-1	3 mg/kg IV every 2 weeks	• Fatigue, rash, vitiligo, pruritus, diarrhea • Immunological toxicities are much less than ipilimumab but possible (hepatotoxicity, endocrinopathies, colitis, skin rash)	• Binds to PD-1 receptor to block PD1 ligands from binding • Prevents the suppression of T cells thereby inducing antitumor immune responses • Clinical response and toxicities take weeks to months to manifest • Manage immunologic toxicities similar to ipilimumab

(*continued*)

95

Agents in the Monoclonal Antibody Class (continued)

Name	FDA-Approved Indication	Target	Dose Range	Toxicities (notable)	Comments
Obinutuzumab (Gazyva™)	Untreated CLL in combination with chlorambucil	CD20	1,000 mg on days 1, 8, and 15 of cycle 1 and on day 1 of cycles 2 through 6 (28-day cycles) (titrate up on first cycle; 100 mg on day 1; 900 mg on day 2)	• Black box warning: HBV reactivation and PML • Infusion-related reactions (generally with first cycle only) • Tumor lysis syndrome (greater risk and infusion reactions than rituximab)	• Premeds: acetaminophen, antihistamine ± corticosteroid • Type 2 monoclonal antibody (does not induce redistribution of CD20 into detergent-resistant lipid rafts) • More direct cytotoxicity and ADCC than rituximab • Less CDC than rituximab • Binds to large loop of CD20 receptor
Ofatumumab (Arzerra®)	CLL	CD20	Untreated: 1,000 mg IV every 28 days × 3–12 cycles (titrate up on first cycle) Refractory: 300 mg week 1, then 2,000 mg weekly × 7 doses, then 2,000 mg q4 weeks (4 doses)	• Infusion-related reactions (generally with first cycle only) • Tumor lysis syndrome • HBV reactivation • PML	• Premeds: acetaminophen, antihistamine ± corticosteroid • Type 1 monoclonal antibody • Similar ADCC and direct cell kill as rituximab • More CDC than rituximab • Binds to small and large loops of CD20 receptor, to an epitope closer to cell membrane

(continued)

Agents in the Monoclonal Antibody Class (*continued*)

Name	FDA-Approved Indication	Target	Dose Range	Toxicities (notable)	Comments
Panitumumab (Vectibix®)	Metastatic colorectal cancer, KRAS WT	EGFR	6 mg/kg every 14 days until disease progression or toxicity	• Black box warning: dermatologic toxicity • Fatigue, skin rash (acneiform, erythema, pruritus), hand-foot syndrome, diarrhea, periungual/nail alterations, hypomagnesemia, nausea, interstitial lung disease, trichomegaly and poliosis of the eyelashes	• Less infusion reactions than cetuximab • Safe option for patients sensitized to galactose-α-1,3-galactose antigen (see cetuximab)
Pembrolizumab (Keytruda®)	Unresectable or metastatic melanoma with progression following ipilimumab and a BRAF inhibitor	PD-1	2 mg/kg every 3 weeks until disease progression or unacceptable toxicity	• Fatigue, rash, vitiligo, pruritus, diarrhea • Immunological toxicities are much less than ipilimumab but possible (hepatotoxicity, endocrinopathies, colitis, skin rash)	• Binds to PD-1 receptor to block PD1 ligands from binding • Prevents the suppression of T cells thereby inducing antitumor immune responses • Clinical response and toxicities take weeks to months to manifest • Manage immunologic toxicities similar to ipilimumab

(*continued*)

Agents in the Monoclonal Antibody Class (*continued*)

Name	FDA-Approved Indication	Target	Dose Range	Toxicities (notable)	Comments
Pertuzumab (Perjeta®)	HER2+ breast cancer (neoadjuvant and metastatic)	HER2	840 mg LD then 420 mg q3 weeks	• Alopecia, rash/hand-foot syndrome, dry skin, fatigue, mucositis, febrile neutropenia, peripheral neuropathy, diarrhea, nausea/vomiting, neutropenia, cardiotoxicity, infusion-related reactions	• Combined with trastuzumab because it binds a different site on the HER2 receptor, preventing HER2 dimerization and leading to a more complete blockade of HER2 signaling • Administer docetaxel after HER2 blockers
Ramucirumab (Cyramza®)	Advanced/metastatic gastric cancer, NSCLC	VEGFR2	8 mg/kg IV every 2 weeks (gastric and colorectal cancer); 10 mg/kg IV every 3 weeks (NSCLC)	• Black box warning: hemorrhage, GI perforation, compromised wound healing • Fistula formation, diarrhea, hypertension, wound dehiscence, peripheral edema, venous and arterial thrombotic effects, proteinuria, infusion-related reactions	• Premeds: H1 antagonist ± dexamethasone and acetaminophen • Specific for VEGF2 receptor • May potentiate concomitant chemotherapy toxicities

(*continued*)

Agents in the Monoclonal Antibody Class (*continued*)

Name	FDA-Approved Indication	Target	Dose Range	Toxicities (notable)	Comments
Rituximab (Rituxan®)	CD20-positive NHLs, CLL in combination with fludarabine and cyclophosphamide	CD20	Initial: 375–500 mg/m² once weekly to every 3 weeks	• Black box warning: infusion-related reactions (generally with first cycle only), mucocutaneous reactions, HBV reactivation, PML • Tumor lysis syndrome, infections, hypogammaglobulinemia	• Premeds: acetaminophen + antihistamine • Type 1 monoclonal antibody • Binds to large loop of CD20 receptor
Tositumomab (Bexxar®) [Antibody-radioisotope conjugate]	Relapsed/refractory CD20+ low-grade, follicular or NHL (failed rituximab)	C20	Requires dosimetry calibration Plts >150,000: 35 mg tositumomab with iodine-131 (I-131) to deliver 75 cGy TBI	• Black box warning: Bone marrow suppression (prolonged and severe), anaphylaxis • Hypothyroidism, infusion reactions, secondary leukemia, fever, rash, nausea, abdominal pain, diarrhea, weakness, myalgia	• Requires thyroid protection • Premeds: acetaminophen, Benadryl • Human anti-mouse antibody + seroconversion (10% of patients) • Antibody-drug conjugate: (a) CD20 antibody, (b) I-131

(*continued*)

Agents in the Monoclonal Antibody Class (*continued*)

Name	FDA-Approved Indication	Target	Dose Range	Toxicities (notable)	Comments
			-Plts <100,000–150,000: 35 mg tositumomab with 65 cGy TBI, single treatment		• Antibody-radioisotope conjugate delivered into cell upon binding to CD20 via endocytosis. Covalent link is hydrolyzed in the acidic environment and I-131 is released. Apoptosis, CDC, ADCC, radiation-induced cell death occur
Trastuzumab (Herceptin®)	HER2+ breast cancer (adjuvant, metastatic), HER2+ metastatic gastric cancer	HER2	4 mg/kg LD, then 2 mg/kg weekly 8 mg/kg LD, then 6 mg/kg every 3 weeks (can also give 6 mg/kg LD and 4 mg/kg every 2 weeks)	• Black box warning: cardiotoxicity: avoid with anthracyclines (generally transient and reversible over 1–3 months), infusion reactions, embryo-fetal toxicity • Pain, headache, nausea/vomiting, diarrhea, infection, pulmonary toxicity	• Not interchangeable with ado-trastuzumab • Adjuvant duration is 52 weeks or 1 year

(continued)

Agents in the Monoclonal Antibody Class (continued)

Name	FDA-Approved Indication	Target	Dose Range	Toxicities (notable)	Comments
Ado-trastuzumab emtansine (Kadcyla®)	HER2 + breast cancer (metastatic patients who have failed trastuzumab and taxane)	HER2	3.6 mg/kg every 3 weeks	• Black box warning: not interchangeable with trastuzumab, cardiotoxicity, hepatotoxicity, embryo-fetal toxicity • Thrombocytopenia (and bleeds), anemia, neutropenia • Hypokalemia, hepatotoxicity, pulmonary toxicity • Fatigue, headache, peripheral neuropathy	• Antibody-drug conjugate: (a) trastuzumab (b) DM1-microtubule inhibitor (maytansine) (c) linker: thioether • Cell cycle arrest in G2/M phase and apoptosis • Maytansine is metabolized by CYP3A4 • An irritant: reactions due to extravasation have been reported

Abbreviations: ADCC, antibody-dependent cell-mediated cytotoxicity; AML, acute myeloid leukemia; APL, acute promyelocytic leukemia; CDC, complement-dependent cytotoxicity; CLL, chronic lymphocytic leukemia; CMV, cytomegalovirus; CTLA-4, cytotoxic T-lymphocyte-associated protein 4; CYP, cytochrome P450; EBV, Epstein–Barr Virus; EGFR, epidermal growth factor receptor; FDA, U.S. Food and Drug Administration; GVHD, graft-versus-host disease; HBV, hepatitis B virus; HER2, human epidermal growth factor receptor type 2; HL, Hodgkin's lymphoma; HUS, hemolytic uremic syndrome; IgE, immunoglobulin E; IV, intravenous; JC virus, John Cunningham virus; LD, loading dose; MDS, myelodysplastic syndrome; MMAE, monomethyl auristatin E; NHL, non-Hodgkin's lymphoma; NSCLC, non-small cell lung cancer; Plt, platelet; PML, progressive multifocal leukoencephalopathy; PNH, paroxysmal nocturnal hemoglobinuria; RANKL, receptor activator of NF kappa B ligand; TBI, total body irradiation; TIW, three times a week; TNF, tumor necrosis factor; VEGF, vascular endothelial growth factor; WBC, white blood cell; WT, wild type; XRT, radiation therapy.

VEGF Trap

What malignancy is ziv-aflibercept approved for?

- Metastatic colorectal cancer

How does ziv-aflibercept work?

- Ziv-aflibercept works by inhibiting angiogenesis, essential for tumor growth

- Ziv-aflibercept is a recombinant fusion protein consisting of portions of the binding domains for vascular endothelial growth factor receptor-1 and -2 (VEGFR1-2), attached to the Fc portion of human immunoglobulin G1 (IgG1), creating a "VEGF Trap" protein

- This fusion protein acts as a decoy receptor for VEGF-A, VEGF-B, and placental growth factor (PIGF), thus preventing VEGFR binding and activation of angiogenesis

What is the usual dose of ziv-aflibercept?

- 4 mg/kg intravenously (IV) over 1 hour every 2 weeks

Is ziv-aflibercept metabolized/eliminated renally or hepatically?

- Ziv-aflibercept is neither metabolized hepatically nor eliminated renally

Are there drug interactions with ziv-aflibercept?

- No clinically important drug-drug interactions have been reported for ziv-aflibercept

What are the most common adverse effects of ziv-aflibercept?

- Headache, fatigue
- Hypertension
- Bleeding
- Gastrointestinal (GI) perforation, fistula formation, and delayed wound healing (all rare but possible)
  - It is recommended to suspend ziv-aflibercept at least 4 weeks prior to surgery and to wait at least 4 weeks after surgery (and after wound has fully healed) to resume therapy
- Proteinuria
- Venous thromboembolism (VTE) and arterial thromboembolic events (transient ischemic attacks [TIAs], cerebrovascular accidents [CVAs], angina, etc.)
- Dysphonia
- Increased liver function tests (LFTs)
- Diarrhea, mucositis
- Hand-foot syndrome, skin hyperpigmentation
- Neutropenia and thrombocytopenia
- Infections

What is the emetogenicity level of ziv-aflibercept?

- Ziv-aflibercept is categorized as low emetic risk (10%–30%)

Is ziv-aflibercept a vesicant or irritant?

- Ziv-aflibercept is neither a vesicant nor an irritant

Tyrosine Kinase Inhibitors

ANGIOGENESIS INHIBITORS AND MULTI-KINASE INHIBITORS

What are the agents in the angiogenesis inhibitor class?

- Sorafenib (Nexavar®), sunitinib (Sutent®), pazopanib (Votrient®), axitinib (Inlyta®), regorafenib (Stivarga®), lenvatinib (Lenvima™), cabozantinib (Cometriq®), vandetanib (Caprelsa®)

What malignancies are each vascular endothelial growth factor receptor (VEGFR) inhibitor FDA approved for?

FDA-Approved Uses of VEGFR Inhibitors

Agent	FDA Approval
Sorafenib	Renal cell carcinoma, hepatocellular carcinoma, thyroid cancer
Sunitinib	Renal cell carcinoma, gastrointestinal stromal tumor, pancreatic neuroendocrine tumors
Pazopanib	Renal cell carcinoma, soft tissue sarcoma
Axitinib	Renal cell carcinoma
Regorafenib	Colorectal cancer (metastatic)
Lenvatinib	Differentiated thyroid cancer (radioactive iodine-refractory)
Cabozantinib	Progressive, metastatic medullary thyroid cancer
Vandetanib	Medullary thyroid cancer, locally advanced or metastatic

Abbreviation: FDA, U.S. Food and Drug Administration.

How do the angiogenesis inhibitors work?

• Vascular endothelial growth factor (VEGF) binds to its receptor tyrosine kinase, VEGFR, to promote angiogenesis and vasculogenesis. VEGFR inhibitors bind intracellularly to the tyrosine kinase, preventing downstream signaling and angiogenesis necessary for tumor growth.

• Platelet-derived growth factor (PDGF) binds to its receptor tyrosine kinase, PDGFR, promoting angiogenesis and activation of various signal transduction pathways leading to proliferation, differentiation, and cell migration. Tyrosine kinase inhibitors of this pathway bind PDGFR intracellularly, preventing this signal transduction and downstream effects.

How do the mechanisms of these tyrosine kinase inhibitors differ?

• Each tyrosine kinase inhibitor has a unique profile of tyrosine kinase targets

Targets for Each Tyrosine Kinase Inhibitor

Agent	Tyrosine Kinase Targets
Sorafenib	VEGFR-1,2,3; PDGFR-β; cKIT; FLT-3; RET; C/BRAF
Sunitinib	VEGFR-1,2,3; PDGFR-α,β; CSF-1R; cKIT; FLT-3; RET
Pazopanib	VEGFR-1,2,3; PDGFR-α,β; FGFR-1,3; cKIT; Itk; c-FMS; Lck
Axitinib	VEGFR-1,2,3
Regorafenib	VEGFR-1,2,3; PDGFR-α,β; FGFR-1,2; TIE2; DDR2; Trk2A; Eph2A; cKIT; RAF-1; BRAF; SAPK2; PTK5; RET; Abl
Lenvatinib	VEGFR-1,2,3; FGFR-1,2,3,4; PDGFR-α; cKIT; RET
Cabozantinib	VEGFR-1,2,3; <u>RET</u>; MET; FLT-3; cKIT; TKRB; AXL; TIE-2
Vandetanib	EGFR; VEGFR; <u>RET</u>; BRK; TIE2; EPH kinase receptors; SRC kinase receptors

- Medullary thyroid cancer is commonly associated with mutations in the rearranged during transfection (RET) proto-oncogene. Thus, cabozantinib and vandetanib, in addition to targeting VEGFR and other key signaling pathways, inhibit RET signaling.

- Gastrointestinal stromal tumor (GIST) is characteristically driven by mutations in cKIT; thus, sunitinib and other agents utilized in GIST (see imatinib in "Breakpoint Cluster Region-Abelson Murine Leukemia Viral Oncogene Homolog 1 [BCR-ABL] Inhibitors") are targeted against inhibition of cKIT signaling.

What are the common dose ranges for each angiogenesis inhibitor?

- Sorafenib: 400 mg orally, twice a day BID (empty stomach)
- Sunitinib: 50 mg orally, daily; 4 weeks on and 2 weeks off, or for some indications, 37.5 mg orally continuous
- Pazopanib: 800 mg orally, daily (empty stomach)
- Axitinib: 5 mg orally, BID (titrate up to 10 mg if no >grade 2 events)
- Regorafenib: 160 mg orally, once daily with food (a low-fat breakfast); 3 weeks on and 1 week off
- Lenvatinib: 24 mg orally, daily
- Cabozantinib: 140 mg orally, daily (empty stomach)
- Vandetanib: 300 mg orally, daily

Are the angiogenesis inhibitors metabolized/eliminated renally or hepatically?

- All eight agents are metabolized hepatically
- Cabozantinib, vandetanib, and lenvatinib require dose adjustments for renal impairment (~25% is eliminated renally)

Are there drug interactions with any of the angiogenesis inhibitors?

- All eight agents have drug interactions with cytochrome P450 inhibitors/inducers

Drug Interactions With Angiogenesis Inhibitors

	CYP1A2	CYP2C8	CYP2C9	CYP2C19	CYP2D6	CYP3A4	UGT1A1	UGT1A9
Sorafenib		INH	INH			SUB	INH	SUB; INH
Sunitinib						SUB		
Pazopanib	SUB	SUB; INH			INH	SUB; INH	INH	
Axitinib	SUB			SUB		SUB	SUB	
Regorafenib						SUB	INH	SUB; INH
Lenvatinib						SUB		
Cabozantinib		SUB				SUB		

Abbreviations: SUB, substrate (bold if major); INH, inhibitor (bold if strong); IND, inducer (bold if strong).

- In vitro, lenvatinib inhibits CYP1A2, 2C8, 2C9, 2C19, 2D6, 3A4, and UGT1A1; however, the clinical significance of this in vitro effect is unknown

- Pazopanib requires an acidic pH for absorption; avoid with agents that raise gastric pH. Consider use of short-acting antacids separated by several hours from administration over longer-acting agents such as proton pump inhibitors (PPIs; suppress acid for ~24 hrs) or H2 receptor antagonists (H2RAs; suppress acid for ~12 hrs)

What are the class adverse effects of the angiogenesis inhibitors?
- Hypertension
- Liver dysfunction
- Rash
- Nausea
- Proteinuria
- Fatigue
- Hair/skin depigmentation
- Hand-foot syndrome
- Delayed wound healing
- Bleeding

- Diarrhea
- Hypothyroidism

What are the most common adverse effects of each angiogenesis inhibitor?

- Sorafenib: hand-foot syndrome, rash, alopecia, hypophosphatemia
- Sunitinib: hand-foot syndrome, mucositis/stomatitis, myelosuppression, dysgeusia, fatigue, hair color changes
- Pazopanib: hypertension, hepatotoxicity, hair color changes
- Axitinib: hypertension, nausea, diarrhea
- Regorafenib: hand-foot skin reaction, fatigue, diarrhea, hypertension, dysphonia, and rash or desquamation
- Lenvatinib: hypertension, diarrhea, fatigue or asthenia, decreased appetite, decreased weight, mucositis, myalgia/arthralgia, dysphonia, and nausea
- Cabozantinib: diarrhea (black box warning for GI perforations, GI fistulas, and GI hemorrhage), rash, hand-foot syndrome, weight loss, decreased appetite, hypertension, increased liver function test (LFTs)
- Vandetanib: diarrhea, QT prolongation (black box warning), restricted access, rash, acne/dermatitis, nausea, hypertension, hypoglycemia

What is the emetogenicity level of the angiogenesis inhibitors?

- All agents are categorized as minimal to low except for lenvatinib
- Lenvatinib is considered moderate to high emetic risk

BREAKPOINT CLUSTER REGION-ABELSON MURINE LEUKEMIA VIRAL ONCOGENE HOMOLOG 1 (BCR-ABL) INHIBITORS

What are the agents in the breakpoint cluster region-Abelson murine leukemia viral oncogene homolog 1 (BCR-ABL) inhibitor class?

- Imatinib (Gleevec®), dasatinib (Sprycel®), nilotinib (Tasigna®), bosutinib (Bosulif®), ponatinib (Iclusig®)

What malignancies are each BCR-ABL inhibitor FDA approved for?

FDA-Approved Uses of BCR-ABL Inhibitors

Agent	FDA Approval
Imatinib	CML (chronic, accelerated, and blast phases), Philadelphia chromosome-positive ALL, myelodysplastic/myeloproliferative disorders with PDGFR gene rearrangements, aggressive systemic mastocytosis (without D816V c-kit mutations), hypereosinophilic syndrome, chronic eosinophilic leukemia with FIP1L1-PDGFRα fusion kinase, dermatofibrosarcoma protuberans, GISTs
Dasatinib	CML (chronic, accelerated, and blast phases)
Nilotinib	CML (chronic and accelerated phases; not blast phase)
Bosutinib	CML (chronic, accelerated, and blast phases)
Ponatinib	CML (chronic, accelerated, and blast phases)

Abbreviations: ALL, acute lymphoblastic leukemia; BCR-ABL, breakpoint cluster region-Abelson murine leukemia viral oncogene homolog 1; CML, chronic myeloid leukemia; FDA, U.S. Food and Drug administration; GIST, gastrointestinal stromal tumor; PDGFR, platelet-derived growth factor receptor.

How do the BCR-ABL inhibitors work in chronic myeloid leukemia (CML)?

- The hallmark genetic driver of CML (and Philadelphia chromosome-positive ALL) is BCR-ABL. ABL is a proto-oncogene that encodes a tyrosine kinase. Upon ABL translocation from chromosome 9 to a position adjacent to BCR on chromosome 22, the resulting BCR-ABL fusion gene produces a BCR-ABL tyrosine kinase that is constitutively active. The overall net effect is leukemogenesis due to constant signaling via the BCR-ABL tyrosine kinase driving cells to divide and proliferate. Cells also lose their ability to undergo apoptosis.

• BCR-ABL inhibitors work by binding to amino acids at the adenosine triphosphate (ATP) binding site of the BCR-ABL tyrosine kinase. This prevents tyrosine kinase autophosphorylation and phosphorylation of downstream signaling pathways that promote leukemogenesis.

• Each BCR-ABL inhibitor binds to the tyrosine kinase differently and with differing potency. Point mutations in the tyrosine kinase lead to resistance to certain BCR-ABL inhibitors.

• The gatekeeper T315I (substitution of a bulky isoleucine residue) mutation blocks access to the ATP binding site, leading to resistance to the majority of tyrosine kinase inhibitors. Ponatinib is structurally designed to contain a carbon-carbon triple bond linkage to avoid steric hindrance from the isoleucine residue, making it the only agent with activity against the T315I mutation.

• Each BCR-ABL inhibitor has multiple other tyrosine kinase targets in addition to BCR-ABL kinase.

What other targets do the BCR-ABL inhibitors have activity against?

• Imatinib: cKIT, PDGFR-α, PDGFR-β, ABL2, CSF1R, SCF

• Dasatinib: SRC family kinases, cKIT, PDGFR-α, PDGFR-β, ABL2, CSF1R (dasatinib inhibits several other kinases)

• Nilotinib: cKIT, PDGFR-α, PDGFR-β, ABL2, CSF1R

• Bosutinib: Src family kinases (does not inhibit cKIT or PDGFR, thus has less myelosuppression)

• Ponatinib: VEGFR-1,2,3, SRC, cKIT, PDGFR-α, PDGFR-β, ABL2, CSF1R (ponatinib inhibits several other kinases)

What are the common dose ranges for each BCR-ABL inhibitor?

• Imatinib: 400 to 600 mg orally, daily (with food); 400 mg orally, BID (with food) for dermatofibrosarcoma protuberans

- Dasatinib: 100 to 140 mg orally, daily
- Nilotinib: 300 to 400 mg orally, BID (empty stomach)
- Bosutinib: 500 to 600 mg orally, daily (with food)
- Ponatinib: 30 to 45 mg orally, daily

Are the BCR-ABL inhibitors metabolized/eliminated renally or hepatically?

- All five agents are metabolized hepatically
- Imatinib requires dose adjustments for renal impairment

Are there drug interactions with any of the BCR-ABL inhibitors?

- All five agents will have drug interactions with cytochrome P450 inhibitors/inducers

Drug Interactions With BCR-ABL Inhibitors

	CYP1A2	CYP2C8	CYP2C9	CYP2C19	CYP2D6	CYP3A4	UGT1A1
Imatinib	SUB	SUB	SUB; INH	SUB	SUB; INH	SUB; INH	
Dasatinib						SUB; INH	
Nilotinib		INH; IND	INH; IND		INH	SUB; INH	INH
Bosutinib						SUB	
Ponatinib		SUB			SUB	SUB	

Abbreviations: BCR-ABL, breakpoint cluster region-Abelson murine leukemia viral oncogene homolog 1; SUB, substrate (bold if major); INH, inhibitor (bold if strong); IND, inducer (bold if strong).

- BCR-ABL inhibitors (with the exception of imatinib) require an acidic pH for absorption; avoid with agents that raise gastric pH. Consider use of short-acting antacids separated by several hours from administration over longer-acting agents such as PPIs (suppress acid for ~24 hrs) or H2RAs (suppress acid for ~12 hrs)

What are the most notable adverse effects of each BCR-ABL inhibitor?

- Imatinib: edema/fluid retention, myalgia, hypophosphatemia, diarrhea, nausea, neutropenia

- Dasatinib: pleural/pericardial effusions, increased bleeding risk, pulmonary arterial hypertension, thrombocytopenia, more neutropenia than imatinib

- Nilotinib: pancreatitis, indirect hyperbilirubinemia (due to inhibition of UGT1A1), hyperglycemia, QT prolongation, peripheral arterial occlusive disease and cardiovascular events, neutropenia

- Bosutinib: diarrhea, nausea/emesis, rash, hepatotoxicity, less myelosuppression than all

- Ponatinib: pancreatitis, hypertension, rash, arterial and venous thrombotic events, hepatotoxicity, more myelosuppression than imatinib

What is the emetogenicity level of the BCR-ABL inhibitors?

- All agents are categorized as minimal to low

B-CELL RECEPTOR (BCR) PATHWAY INHIBITORS

What are the agents in the B-cell receptor (BCR) pathway inhibitor class?

- Ibrutinib (Imbruvica®)
- Idelalisib (Zydelig®)

What malignancies are each BCR pathway inhibitor FDA approved for?

FDA-Approved Uses of BCR Pathway Inhibitors

Agent	FDA Approval
Ibrutinib	Mantle cell lymphoma (MCL), chronic lymphocytic leukemia (CLL), Waldenström's macroglobulinemia (WM)
Idelalisib	CLL (in combination with rituximab), follicular lymphoma, small lymphocytic lymphoma

Abbreviations: BCR, B-cell receptor; FDA, U.S. Food and Drug Administration.

How do the BCR pathway inhibitors work? (Figure 8.1)

- The BCR is composed of membrane immunoglobulins associated with Igα and Igβ heterodimers (CD79a/CD79b). The membrane immunoglobulins bind antigen extracellularly and activate the heterodimers; intracellular signal transduction results
- Antigen- or ligand-independent signaling also occurs (tonic signaling)
- Both antigen-dependent and antigen-independent signaling lead to activation of the Src family kinases, Syk, Bruton's tyrosine kinase (BTK), phospholipase C (PLCγ2), phosphoinositide 3-kinase (PI3K), and other signaling molecules and cascades
- As a result, many cellular processes occur, such as differentiation, proliferation, motility, homing, adhesion, chemotaxis, and survival

How do the mechanisms of ibrutinib and idelalisib differ? (Figure 8.1)

- Ibrutinib: BTK inhibitor (although also has several other targets)

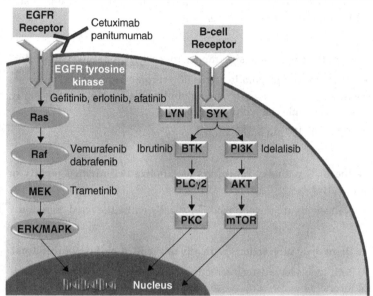

FIGURE 8.1. Tyrosine kinase and monoclonals: Mutations in epidermal growth factor receptor (EGFR) and BRAF lead to hyperstimulation of the EGFR-Ras-Raf-MEK-ERK/MAPK pathway resulting in hyperproliferation, reduced apoptosis, and increased invasiveness/metastatic potential of cancer cells. Monoclonal antibodies bind to receptors extracellularly. Cetuximab and panitumumab bind to the EGFR receptor and block downstream signal transduction. Tyrosine kinase inhibitors act intracellularly to inhibit tyrosine kinase signaling. The tyrosine kinase inhibitors gefitinib, erlotinib, and afatinib bind and inhibit the EGFR tyrosine kinase, preventing phosphorylation and thereby inhibiting further downstream signaling. Vemurafenib and dabrafenib bind and inhibit the BRAF kinase preventing phosphorylation and thereby inhibiting further downstream signaling. Trametinib binds and inhibits MEK, which is downstream of BRAF. The B-cell receptor is activated by both antigen-dependent and antigen-independent signaling. Overactivation of the Src family kinases (Lyn and Syk), BTK, PLCγ2, PI3K, and other signaling molecules and cascades can occur in various lymphomas/leukemias. As a result, many cellular processes occur such as proliferation, motility, homing, adhesion, chemotaxis, and survival. Ibrutinib inhibits BTK and idelalisib inhibits PI3K-δ.

- Idelalisib: phosphoinositide 3-kinase delta (PI3Kδ) kinase inhibitor (although also has several other targets)

What are the common dosing ranges for each BCR pathway inhibitor?

- Ibrutinib: 420 mg orally, daily (for chronic lymphocytic leukemia [CLL] and Waldenström's macroglobulinemia [WM]); 560 mg orally, daily (for mantle cell lymphoma [MCL])
- Idelalisib: 150 mg orally, BID

Are the BCR pathway inhibitors metabolized/eliminated renally or hepatically?

- Both agents are metabolized hepatically with little renal excretion

Are there drug interactions with any of the BCR pathway inhibitors?

- Both agents have drug interactions with cytochrome P450 inhibitors/inducers

Drug Interactions With BCR Pathway Inhibitors

	CYP1A2	CYP2C8	CYP2C9	CYP2C19	CYP2D6	CYP3A4	UGT1A1	UGT1A4
Ibrutinib						SUB		
Idelalisib	INH		INH			SUB; INH	INH	SUB

Abbreviations: INH, inhibitor (bold if strong); SUB, substrate (bold if major).

- Ibrutinib should be avoided in patients on warfarin due to bleeding risk from the antiplatelet effect of ibrutinib; ibrutinib should also be used with caution in those taking other therapeutic anticoagulants or antiplatelet drugs, as bleeding risk can increase significantly
- While systemic ibrutinib is unlikely to inhibit P-glycoprotein (P-gp), higher local concentrations in the GI tract may lead to an effect on P-gp substrates in the GI tract. Use caution when coadministering ibrutinib with substrates of P-gp with a narrow therapeutic index (eg, digoxin)

What are the most notable adverse effects of each BCR pathway inhibitor?

- Ibrutinib: diarrhea, bruising, rash, petechiae, bleeding, atrial fibrillation, lymphocytosis, neutropenia

- Idelalisib: diarrhea (early and late onset; late onset is thought to be an immune-mediated colitis), pyrexia, fatigue, neutropenia, rash, hepatotoxicity, pneumonitis, intestinal perforation

What is the emetogenicity level of the BCR pathway inhibitors?

- Both agents are considered minimal to low risk

EGFR-RAS-RAF-MEK-ERK (MAPK) PATHWAY INHIBITORS

What are the agents in the mitogen-activated protein kinase (MAPK) pathway inhibitor class?

- Epidermal growth factor receptor (EGFR) inhibitors—gefitinib (Iressa®), erlotinib (Tarceva®), afatinib (Gilotrif™)

- BRAF inhibitors—vemurafenib (Zelboraf®), dabrafenib (Tafinlar®)

- MEK inhibitor—trametinib (Mekinist™)

What malignancies are each MAPK pathway inhibitor FDA approved for?

FDA-Approved Uses of MAPK Pathway Inhibitors

Agent	FDA Approval
Gefitinib	Non–small cell lung cancer (NSCLC)
Erlotinib	NSCLC, pancreatic cancer
Afatinib	NSCLC
Vemurafenib	Melanoma (BRAF mutated)
Dabrafenib	Melanoma (BRAF mutated) single agent and in combination with trametinib
Trametinib	Melanoma (BRAF mutated)

Abbreviations: FDA, U.S. Food and Drug Administration; MAPK, mitogen-activated protein kinase.

How do the MAPK pathway inhibitors work? (Figure 8.1)

- Mutations in the EGFR and BRAF tyrosine kinases lead to hyperstimulation of the EGFR-Ras-Raf-MEK-ERK pathway resulting in hyperproliferation, reduced apoptosis, and increased invasiveness/metastatic potential

- Gefitinib, erlotinib, and afatinib bind and inhibit the EGFR tyrosine kinase, preventing phosphorylation of downstream targets, thereby inhibiting further MAPK pathway signaling

- Vemurafenib and dabrafenib bind and inhibit the BRAF kinase, preventing phosphorylation of downstream targets, thereby inhibiting further MAPK signaling

- Trametinib binds to and inhibits MEK, which is downstream of BRAF

What are the common dose ranges for each MAPK pathway inhibitor?

- Gefitinib: 250 mg orally, daily

- Erlotinib: 150 mg orally, daily (non–small cell lung cancer [NSCLC]); 100 mg orally, daily (pancreatic; empty stomach)

- Afatinib: 40 mg orally, daily (empty stomach)

- Vemurafenib: 960 mg orally, BID

- Dabrafenib: 150 mg orally, BID (empty stomach)

- Trametinib: 2 mg orally, daily (empty stomach)

Are the MAPK pathway inhibitors metabolized/eliminated renally or hepatically?

- Gefitinib, erlotinib, vemurafenib, and dabrafenib are metabolized hepatically

- Afatinib does not require renal or hepatic adjustments; this agent is covalently adducted to proteins and nucleophilic small molecules and eliminated in feces

- Trametinib does not require renal or hepatic adjustments; this agent is deacetylated by hydrolytic enzymes (carboxylesterases or amidases) and eliminated in feces

Are there drug interactions with any of the MAPK pathway inhibitors?

- Gefitinib, erlotinib, vemurafenib, and dabrafenib have drug interactions with cytochrome P450 inhibitors/inducers

Drug Interactions With MAPK Pathway Inhibitors

	CYP1A2	CYP2C8	CYP2C9	CYP2C19	CYP2D6	CYP3A4	UGT1A1
Gefitinib				INH	SUB; INH	SUB	
Erlotinib	SUB					SUB	
Afatinib							
Vemurafenib	INH				INH	SUB; IND	
Dabrafenib		SUB; IND	IND	IND		SUB; IND	IND
Trametinib							

Abbreviations: IND, inducer (bold if strong); INH, inhibitor (bold if strong); SUB, substrate (bold if major).

- Gefitinib, erlotinib, and dabrafenib require an acidic pH for absorption; avoid with agents that raise gastric pH. Consider use of short-acting antacids separated by several hours from administration over longer-acting agents such as PPIs (suppress acid for ~24 hrs) or H2RAs (suppress acid for ~12 hrs)

- Afatinib and dabrafenib: P-gp substrates/inhibitors/inducers (afatinib and dabrafenib are both substrates and inhibitors of P-gp)

What are the most common adverse effects of each MAPK pathway inhibitor?

- Gefitinib: rash, diarrhea, stomatitis, alopecia, pruritus, dry skin, conjunctivitis, paronychia; also monitor for pneumonitis, hepatotoxicity, GI perforation, ocular disorders (inflammation, blurred vision, eye pain, lacrimation, light sensitivity, keratitis)

- Erlotinib: similar toxicity profile as gefitinib (possibly increased rash, fatigue, stomatitis, anorexia, less diarrhea, and less nail changes compared with gefitinib)

- Afatinib: diarrhea (more than erlotinib/gefitinib), rash, acne, stomatitis, paronychia, dry skin, pruritus, epistaxis, cheilitis; also monitor for pneumonitis, hepatotoxicity, GI perforation, and ocular toxicities

- Vemurafenib: arthralgia, rash, fatigue, photosensitivity, cutaneous squamous cell carcinoma, QT prolongation, hepatotoxicity

- Dabrafenib: hand-foot syndrome, pyrexia, hyperglycemia, hypophosphatemia; the following adverse effects occur but at a lower rate than with vemurafenib: rash, photosensitivity, squamous cell carcinoma, arthralgia

- Trametinib: rash, diarrhea, peripheral edema, fatigue, dermatitis acneiform, decreased ejection fraction, ocular disorders (blurred vision)

What is the emetogenicity level of the MAPK pathway inhibitors?

- All agents are considered minimal to low risk

MISCELLANEOUS ORAL TARGETED THERAPIES

What are the agents in the category?

- Ruxolitinib (Jakafi™), crizotinib (Xalkori®), ceritinib (Zykadia™), lapatinib (Tykerb®), palbociclib (Ibrance®), olaparib (Lynparza™), vismodegib (Erivedge™), sonidegib (Odomzo®)

What malignancies are each agent FDA approved for?

FDA-Approved Uses of Miscellaneous Oral Targeted Therapies

Agent	FDA Approval
Ruxolitinib	Myelofibrosis, polycythemia vera
Crizotinib	Myelofibrosis, polycythemia vera
Ceritinib	Myelofibrosis, polycythemia vera
Lapatinib	Breast cancer (in combination with capecitabine or letrozole)
Palbociclib	Breast cancer (in combination with letrozole)
Olaparib	Ovarian cancer (with suspected or proven germline BRCA mutation)
Vismodegib	Basal cell carcinoma
Sonidegib	Basal cell carcinoma

Abbreviation: FDA, U.S. Food and Drug Administration.

How do these agents work?

- Ruxolitinib: Janus Kinases (JAKs) are nonreceptor tyrosine kinases that mediate signaling of cytokines and growth factors responsible for hematopoiesis. JAK stimulates signal transducers and activators of transcription (STATs), which leads to gene expression. Aberrant activation of the JAK/STAT pathway is implicated in a number of disease states. JAK2-V617F mutations, other point mutations, excess cytokines, and other aberrations lead to dysregulated JAK signaling, ultimately resulting in myelofibrosis. Ruxolitinib inhibits JAK1 and JAK2 (the presence of the JAK2-V617F mutation specifically is not required for activity).

• Crizotinib and ceritinib: Anaplastic lymphoma receptor tyrosine kinase (ALK) is a transmembrane protein and echinoderm microtubule-associated protein like 4 (EML4) is a cytoplasmic protein involved in microtubule formation. ALK and EML4 reside in close proximity on chromosome 2. An intrachromosomal rearrangement can occur, resulting in the juxtaposition of ALK and EML4 creating a fusion protein. The EML4-ALK fusion protein leads to constitutive activation of downstream signal transduction pathways leading to the hyperproliferation of cells and inhibition of apoptosis. Crizotinib and ceritinib both bind to and inhibit the EML4-ALK fusion protein. ALK also may have other fusion partners that lead to oncogenesis (eg, NPM-ALK in anaplastic large cell lymphoma).

– Crizotinib also inhibits c-ros oncogene 1 (ROS1), hepatocyte growth factor receptor (HGFR)/mesenchymal epithelial transition growth factor (c-MET), and recepteur d'origine nantais (RON)

– Ceritinib also inhibits insulin-like growth factor 1 receptor (IGF-1R), insulin receptor (InsR), and ROS1

• Lapatinib: In human epidermal receptor type 2 (HER2)+ breast cancer, the HER2 gene is amplified increasing the expression of the HER2 tyrosine kinase receptor. Several phenotypic consequences result from HER2 overexpression such as increased proliferation and survival, increased mutagenesis, increased metastatic potential and cellular motility, and increased secretion of growth factors. Lapatinib is an inhibitor of the intracellular tyrosine kinase domains of both EGFR and the HER2 receptor.

• Palbociclib: Many signal transduction pathways converge at the level of cyclinD1. CyclinD1 activates cyclin-dependent kinase (CDK4/6) and the two form a complex. This complex phosphorylates the retinoblastoma (RB) tumor suppressor protein, which inactivates the RB protein. Normally, RB inhibits E2F (a transcription factor) from interacting with the cell's transcription machinery. However, RB protein inactivation by the complex results in the release of E2F transcription factors, which allows for continuous cell cycle progression from the G1 phase to S phase. Palbociclib competitively blocks CDK4/6 from binding and forming a complex with cyclinD1, thus preventing continuous cell cycle progression.

• Olaparib: Poly ADP ribose polymerase (PARP) is a DNA repair enzyme responsible for repairing single-strand DNA breaks. During DNA replication, single-strand breaks occur. If unrepaired, collision of the replication fork with the lesion produces a double-strand DNA break. Several mechanisms of DNA repair exist to restore double-strand breaks. One such mechanism is homologous recombination. Normal cells have intact homologous recombination; however, a subset of tumor cells are deficient in homologous recombination. The most notable deficiencies occur in tumors with breast cancer type susceptibility protein 1 or 2 (BRCA1 and/or BRCA2) mutations. Inhibition of PARP with olaparib prevents single-strand DNA repair, which leads to double-strand DNA breaks upon collision of the replication fork. In normal cells, homologous recombination repairs the double-strand DNA breaks. However, in tumor cells with deficiencies in homologous recombination repair pathways (such as BRCA1/2), repair of double-strand breaks cannot occur, resulting in the accumulation of defective DNA lesions. Ultimately, cessation of DNA synthesis and apoptosis occurs.

• Vismodegib and sonidegib: The hedgehog pathway has several key components: the hedgehog ligand (hedgehog), the hedgehog receptor (patched), the cell surface signal transducer (smoothened), and its downstream effector (GLI transcription factors). In the absence of the hedgehog ligand, Patched normally inhibits Smoothened, preventing activation of downstream signaling via GLI transcription factors. Mutations can occur in Patched (the inhibitory receptor) or Smoothened, both inducing aberrant activation of downstream signaling to GLI and thus increasing expression of various genes that promote cell proliferation and differentiation.

What are the common dose ranges for each agent?

• Ruxolitinib: Starting dose for myelofibrosis is based on the patient's baseline platelet count (20 mg orally BID, 15 mg orally BID, or 5 mg orally BID for platelets of 200, 100, and 50×10^9/L, respectively); 10 mg orally, BID for polycythemia vera

• Crizotinib: 250 mg orally, BID

• Ceritinib: 750 mg orally, daily (empty stomach)

- Lapatinib: 1,250 mg orally, daily (empty stomach) when in combination with capecitabine; 1,500 mg orally, daily (empty stomach) when in combination with letrozole

- Palbociclib: 125 mg orally, daily (with food); 21 days on, 7 days off

- Olaparib: 400 mg orally, BID

- Vismodegib: 150 mg orally, daily

- Sonidegib: 200 mg orally, daily (empty stomach)

Are these agents metabolized/eliminated renally or hepatically?

- All agents are metabolized hepatically

- Ruxolitinib is also eliminated renally

Are there drug interactions with any of these agents?

- All drugs except vismodegib will have drug interactions with cytochrome P450 inhibitors/inducers (although vismodegib is a CYP substrate, CYP inhibitors are not predicted to alter its systemic concentrations)

Drug Interactions With Miscellaneous Oral Targeted Therapies

	CYP1A2	CYP2C8	CYP2C9	CYP2C19	CYP2D6	CYP3A4	UGT1A1
Ruxolitinib						SUB	
Crizotinib						SUB; INH	
Ceritinib				INH		SUB; INH	
Lapatinib		INH				SUB; INH	
Palbociclib						SUB; INH	
Olaparib						SUB	
Vismodegib	INH	SUB; INH	INH			SUB	
Sonidegib		INH				SUB	

Abbreviations: IND, inducer (bold if strong); INH, inhibitor (bold if strong); SUB, substrate (bold if major).

- Crizotinib, ceritinib, lapatinib, and vismodegib are P-gp substrates; crizotinib and lapatinib are inhibitors of P-gp. Crizotinib, ceritinib, lapatinib, vismodegib, palbociclib, and sonidegib concentrations can be reduced with the coadministration of antacids

What are the most common adverse effects of each agent?

- Ruxolitinib: anemia, thrombocytopenia, neutropenia, ecchymosis, dizziness, headache, pyrexia, hypercholesterolemia
- Crizotinib: nausea/vomiting, diarrhea, ocular toxicities, hepatotoxicity, pneumonitis, hypogonadism, QT prolongation
- Ceritinib: nausea/vomiting, diarrhea (more severe than crizotinib), hepatotoxicity, hyperglycemia, hypophosphatemia, anemia, increased lipase levels
- Lapatinib: reduced ejection fraction (appears to be less than trastuzumab), rash, hand-foot syndrome, dry skin, diarrhea (generally within 6 days and duration of 4–5 days), fatigue, QT prolongation, hepatotoxicity (patients who carry the human leukocyte antigen [HLA] alleles DQA1*02:01 and DRV1*07:01 may be at greater risk)
- Palbociclib: neutropenia, leukopenia, fatigue, stomatitis, anemia, thrombocytopenia, neuropathy
- Olaparib: anemia, nausea/vomiting, dyspnea, arthralgia, myalgia, rash, increased serum creatinine, dysgeusia
- Vismodegib: nausea/vomiting, diarrhea, muscle spasms, arthralgia, alopecia, dysgeusia, possibility for promotion of cutaneous squamous cell carcinoma
- Sonidegib: Elevations in creatine kinase and lipase, hyperglycemia, increased LFTs, muscle spasms and myalgia, alopecia, dysgeusia, nausea, fatigue, weight loss, diarrhea, pruritus, possibility for promotion of cutaneous squamous cell carcinoma

What is the emetogenicity level of these agents?

- Crizotinib, ceritinib, olaparib, and vismodegib are considered moderate to high

- All other agents are considered minimal to low
- Sonidegib has not been assigned a category at the time of writing; however, this agent likely fits within the moderate to high category

9

Antiandrogen Therapies

What are the agents in the antiandrogen class?

- Abiraterone (Zytiga®) and enzalutamide (Xtandi®)

What malignancies are each antiandrogen FDA approved for?

FDA-Approved Uses of Antiandrogen Therapies

Agent	FDA Approval
Abiraterone	Prostate cancer
Enzalutamide	Prostate cancer

Abbreviation: FDA, U.S. Food and Drug Administration.

How do the antiandrogens work?

- Abiraterone: inhibits the 17 α-hydroxylase/C17,20-lyase enzyme required for androgen biosynthesis (expressed in testicular, adrenal, and prostate tumor tissues); inhibits formations of the testosterone precursors, dehydroepiandrosterone (DHEA) and androstenedione

  – Due to the inhibition of steroid synthesis by abiraterone, this agent must be taken with prednisone (see the following text) in order to avoid mineralocorticoid excess (caused by a rise in adrenocorticotropic hormone [ACTH] via a positive feedback loop) and consequences of low cortisol

- Enzalutamide: a pure androgen receptor inhibitor which, unlike traditional antiandrogens (eg, bicalutamide, flutamide), does not exhibit agonist properties upon binding to the androgen receptor. Enzalutamide binds to the androgen receptor with much higher affinity than traditional antiandrogens, prevents nuclear translocation of the androgen receptor, and prevents androgen receptor association with DNA

What are the common dose ranges for each antiandrogen?

- Abiraterone: 1,000 mg orally daily (empty stomach) with prednisone 5 mg orally (PO) BID
- Enzalutamide: 160 mg orally once daily (with or without food)

Are the antiandrogens metabolized/eliminated renally or hepatically?

- Both agents are metabolized hepatically
- Enzalutamide is also renally eliminated (primarily as inactive metabolites)

Are there drug interactions with any of the antiandrogens?

- Abiraterone: CYP3A4 inhibitors/inducers; spironolactone (activates the androgen receptor); abiraterone inhibits CYP2C8/2C19/2C9/2D6/3A4
- Enzalutamide: a CYP2C8 and 3A4 substrate—reduce dose (80 mg) with strong CYP2C8 inhibitors; enzalutamide is an inducer of CYP3A4, CYP2C9, and CYP2C19

What are the adverse effects of each agent?

- Abiraterone: fluid retention/edema, hypokalemia, hypertension, cardiac disorders (ischemic heart disease, myocardial infarction, arrhythmias, heart failure), hepatotoxicity, hot flushes
- Enzalutamide: asthenia/fatigue is the most common side effect; arthralgia, hot flushes, hypertension, seizures are rare

What is the emetogenicity level of the antiandrogens?

- These agents are not chemotherapy and therefore are not in the National Comprehensive Cancer Network (NCCN) categorization; emetogenicity is minimal to low

10

Mammalian Target of Rapamycin (mTOR) Inhibitors

What are the agents in the mTOR inhibitor class?

- Everolimus (Afinitor®) and temsirolimus (Torisel®)

What malignancies are each mTOR inhibitor FDA approved for?

FDA-Approved Uses of mTOR Inhibitors

Agent	FDA Approval
Everolimus	Renal cell carcinoma, breast cancer (in combination with letrozole or anastrozole), primitive neuroectodermal tumor (PNET)
Temsirolimus	Renal cell carcinoma

Abbreviations: FDA, U.S. Food and Drug Administration; mTOR, mammalian target of rapamycin.

How do the mTOR inhibitors work?

- The PI3K/AKT/mTOR pathway is dysregulated in various malignancies, leading to uncontrolled cell growth, proliferation, motility, and survival. This pathway can also become constitutively activated as a mechanism for resistance

- The mTOR inhibitors first bind to the FK binding protein 12 (FKBP-12). This complex binds to the mTOR complex 1 (mTORc1) and inhibits downstream signaling of the PI3K/AKT/mTOR pathway

What are the common dose ranges for each mTOR inhibitor?

- Everolimus: 10 mg orally, daily
- Temsirolimus: 25 mg intravenous, weekly

Are the mTOR inhibitors metabolized/eliminated renally or hepatically?

- Both agents are metabolized hepatically

Are there drug interactions with any of the mTOR inhibitors?

- Everolimus and temsirolimus are substrates of CYP3A4 and P-glycoprotein (P-gp); thus, inhibitors/inducers of this enzyme and transporter may increase or decrease levels, respectively. Of note, one of the metabolites of temsirolimus is sirolimus, an active metabolite also metabolized by CYP3A4.

What are the major adverse effects of the mTOR inhibitors?

- Hyperlipidemia
- Hyperglycemia
- Dyspnea and pneumonitis
- Mucositis, stomatitis, and diarrhea
- Edema
- Rash, pruritus
- Decreased wound healing
- Infections due to increased immunosuppression
- Hypophosphatemia
- Hypertriglyceridemia

What is the emetogenicity level of the mTOR inhibitors?

- Everolimus is categorized as minimal to low emetic risk
- Temsirolimus is categorized as minimal emetic risk

Histone Deacetylase (HDAC) Inhibitors

What are the chemotherapy agents in the HDAC inhibitor class?

- Vorinostat (Zolinza®), romidepsin (Istodax®), belinostat (Beleodaq®), panobinostat (Farydaq®)

What malignancies are each HDAC inhibitor approved for?

FDA-Approved Uses of HDAC Inhibitors

Agent	FDA Approval
Vorinostat	Cutaneous T-cell lymphoma (CTCL)
Romidepsin	CTCL, peripheral T-cell lymphoma (PTCL)
Belinostat	PTCL
Panobinostat	Multiple myeloma

Abbreviations: FDA, U.S. Food and Drug Administration; HDAC, histone deacetylase.

How do the HDAC inhibitors work?

- HDAC is an enzyme that catalyzes the removal of acetyl groups from histones. By removing acetyl groups, DNA wraps more tightly around histones, preventing gene expression of tumor suppressor genes

- HDAC inhibitors bind to this enzyme and inhibit its function, leading to increased acetylation of DNA and expression of previously silenced genes

- Ultimately, reactivated gene effects lead to cell cycle arrest and apoptosis

• In patients with multiple myeloma, panobinostat and other HDAC inhibitors act synergistically with proteasome inhibitors. Proteasome inhibitors lead to the accumulation of ubiquitinated protein aggregates, which contribute to cell death. Ubiquitinated proteins can be alternatively degraded by the aggresome pathway, which is dependent on HDAC6. Inhibition of HDAC6 by HDAC inhibitors leads to synergistic cytotoxicity of myeloma cells in combination with proteasome inhibitors.

What are the common mechanisms of resistance to HDAC inhibitor therapy?

• Romidepsin, belinostat, and panobinostat are substrates for P-glycoprotein (P-gp). Increased P-gp expression can increase active drug efflux from malignant cells

• Overexpression of antiapoptotic proteins, such as BCL-2 or BCL-X$_L$

• Overexpression and increased activation of the Jak/STAT pathway

What are the common dosing ranges for each HDAC inhibitor?

• Vorinostat: 400 mg orally (PO) once daily with food

• Romidepsin: 14 mg/m^2 intravenous (IV) on days 1, 8, and 15 of a 28-day cycle

• Belinostat: 1,000 mg/m^2 IV daily × 5 days of a 21-day cycle

  – Patients homozygous for the UGT1A1*28 allele have significantly reduced UGT1A1 activity (responsible for the metabolism of belinostat) and require a lower starting dose of belinostat (750 mg/m^2)

• Panobinostat: 20 mg PO every other day for three doses each week for 2 weeks of a 21-day cycle (days 1, 3, 5, 8, 10, and 12)

Are the HDAC inhibitors metabolized/eliminated renally or hepatically?

• The HDAC inhibitors are all metabolized hepatically and require dose adjustment for hepatic dysfunction

Are there drug interactions with any of the HDAC inhibitors?

- All HDAC inhibitors: additional QTc prolonging agents

- Vorinostat: warfarin (increases in international normalized ratio [INR] have been documented)

- Romidepsin: modulators of the CYP3A4 pathway (responsible for romidepsin metabolism), warfarin (increases in INR have been documented)

- Belinostat: inhibitors or inducers of UGT1A1

- Panobinostat: modulators of the CYP3A4 pathway (responsible for the metabolism of panobinostat); drugs metabolized through CYP2D6 (panobinostat inhibits CYP2D6)

What are the most common adverse effects of the HDAC inhibitors?

- EKG changes (including QTc prolongation)

- Nausea, vomiting, dysgeusia, diarrhea

- Mild myelosuppression (typically more thrombocytopenia and anemia)

What is the emetogenicity level of the HDAC inhibitors?

- All six agents are categorized as low (10%–30% frequency)

Are the HDAC inhibitors vesicants or irritants?

- The HDAC inhibitors are neither vesicants nor irritants

Hypomethylating Agents

What are the chemotherapy agents in the hypomethylating agent class?

- Azacitidine (Vidaza®), decitabine (Dacogen®)

What malignancies are each hypomethylating agent FDA approved for?

- Both are approved for the treatment of myelodysplastic syndrome (MDS)

How do the hypomethylating agents work? (Figure 12.1)

- Summary: Hypomethylating agents are epigenetic modifiers, which cause global DNA hypomethylation, resulting in the transcription of previously aberrantly silenced genes such as tumor suppressor genes

- Azacitidine and decitabine are cytidine nucleoside analogues that are incorporated into DNA and RNA as false base pairs

  – Azacitidine has a greater propensity to incorporate into RNA, while decitabine is exclusively incorporated into DNA

- After incorporation into DNA, azacitidine and decitabine inhibit DNA methyltransferase, the epigenetic enzyme responsible for adding methyl groups to DNA bases and preventing gene transcription

- Previously methylated and silenced genes including tumor suppressor genes and those that control cancer cell differentiation are expressed

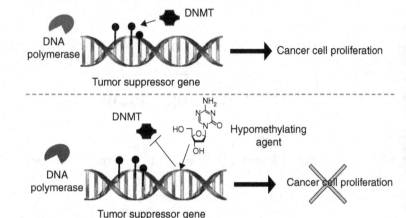

FIGURE 12.1. Hypomethylating agent MOA: The hypomethylating agents, azacitidine and decitabine, are cytidine analogues that are incorporated into DNA and inhibit DNA methyltransferase (DNMT). DNMT is an enzyme responsible for the epigenetic modification of DNA base pairs via methylation. This methylation of DNA prevents transcription of genes critical for tumor suppression and differentiation. By inhibiting DNMT, DNA becomes globally hypomethylated, and these genes are expressed, preventing tumor cell proliferation.

What are the common dosing ranges for the hypomethylating agents?

- Azacitidine: 75 mg/m^2 subcutaneous/intravenous (IV) daily × 7 days every 28 days

- Decitabine: 20 mg/m^2 IV daily × 5 to 10 days every 28 days

Are the hypomethylating agents metabolized/eliminated renally or hepatically?

- Azacitidine and decitabine are primarily metabolized by cytidine deaminase, and azacitidine is eliminated renally; however, initial dosage adjustments for renal or hepatic impairment are generally not required for either agent

Are there drug interactions with any of the hypomethylating agents?

- No clinically significant drug interactions exist for the hypomethylating agents

What are the most common adverse effects of the hypomethylating agents?

- Myelosuppression
- Fever
- Fatigue
- Diarrhea/constipation

What is the emetogenicity level of the hypomethylating agents?

- The National Comprehensive Cancer Network (NCCN) characterizes azacitidine as moderate (30%–90% frequency)
- Decitabine has minimal emetogenic potential (<10% frequency)

Are the hypomethylating agents vesicants or irritants?

- Decitabine and azacitidine are neither vesicants nor irritants

Proteasome Inhibitors

What are the chemotherapy agents in the proteasome inhibitor class?

- Bortezomib (Velcade®), carfilzomib (Kyprolis®)

What malignancies are each proteasome inhibitor FDA approved for?

FDA-Approved Uses of Proteasome Inhibitors

Bortezomib	Carfilzomib
Multiple myeloma, mantle cell lymphoma	Multiple myeloma, relapsed/ refractory

Abbreviation: FDA, U.S. Food and Drug Administration.

How do the proteasome inhibitors work?

- In normal cells, the proteasome works to degrade intracellular proteins and maintain homeostasis

- Proteasome inhibitors bind and inhibit the chymotrypsin-like activity of the proteasome, preventing degradation of intracellular proteins

  – Bortezomib binds reversibly to the proteasome

  – Carfilzomib binds irreversibly, is more potent than bortezomib, more selective for the chymotrypsin-like activity of the proteasome, and is active in bortezomib-resistant cells

- Accumulation of proteins normally marked for degradation leads to cell death through the unfolded protein response and the endoplasmic reticulum stress pathway

• Accumulation of proteins critical for regulating cell cycle progression (eg, p27, cyclin B) leads to cell cycle arrest

• Proteasome inhibitors also inhibit nuclear factor kappa B (NF-KB) activity of cancer cells through preventing degradation of the inhibitor of NF-KB (IKB); NF-KB activation is heavily involved in cell proliferation, angiogenesis, and suppression of apoptosis

What are the common mechanisms of resistance to proteasome inhibitor therapy?

• Alternative degradation of ubiquitinated proteins through the aggresome pathway, dependent on histone deacetylase 6 (HDAC6) (HDAC inhibitors can synergize with proteasome inhibitors through inhibition of this resistance pathway—see Chapter 11)

• Mutations in the β-subunits of the proteasome that alter proteasome inhibitor binding

• Upregulation of proteasomal subunits

What are the common dosing ranges for each proteasome inhibitor?

• Bortezomib: 1.3 mg/m^2 intravenously (IV)/subcutaneously (subQ) days 1, 4, 8, and 11 of a 21-day cycle; 1.5 mg/m^2 IV weekly, days 1, 8, 15, and 22 of a 28-day cycle

• Carfilzomib: 20 mg/m^2 IV days 1, 2, 8, 9, 15, and 16 (cycle 1; 28-day cycle), then 27 mg/m^2 IV days 1, 2, 8, 9, 15, and 16 of subsequent 28-day cycles

Are the proteasome inhibitors metabolized/eliminated renally or hepatically?

• The proteasome inhibitors are metabolized hepatically and require dose adjustment for hepatic dysfunction

Are there drug interactions with any of the proteasome inhibitors?

• Drugs that modulate the CYP3A4 pathway may increase/decrease bortezomib concentrations

What are the most common adverse effects of the proteasome inhibitors?

- Peripheral neuropathy
  - Typically a reversible sensory neuropathy
  - More common with bortezomib than carfilzomib
  - SubQ administration and weekly administration of bortezomib have both been shown (individually) to reduce peripheral neuropathy without impacting efficacy
- Myelosuppression (primarily thrombocytopenia)
- Herpes zoster and herpes simplex reactivation (prophylaxis with acyclovir is recommended)
- Nausea, vomiting, and diarrhea (typically mild)
- Fevers, fatigue, and weakness
- Congestive heart failure, dyspnea, peripheral edema, and renal failure (more common with carfilzomib)

What are the premedications required?

Premedications Required for Proteasome Inhibitors

Drug	Premedication
Bortezomib	None
Carfilzomib	250–500 mL normal saline (or other intravenous [IV] fluid) predose; can also give another 250–500 mL postdose if needed
	Dexamethasone 4 mg (oral or IV) prior to all doses in cycle 1, all doses with dose escalation cycle, and as needed with future cycles to reduce infusion reaction risk

What is the emetogenicity level of the proteasome inhibitors?

- Both agents are categorized as low (10%–30% frequency)

Are the proteasome inhibitors vesicants or irritants?

- Bortezomib and carfilzomib are neither vesicants nor irritants

Immunomodulatory Agents

What are the chemotherapy agents in the immunomodulatory agent (IMiD) class?

- Thalidomide (Thalomid®), lenalidomide (Revlimid®), pomalidomide (Pomalyst®)

What malignancies are the IMiDs FDA approved for?

FDA-Approved Uses of Immunomodulatory Agents (IMiDs)

Agent	FDA Approval
Thalidomide	Multiple myeloma
Lenalidomide	Multiple myeloma, mantle cell lymphoma, myelodysplastic syndrome (with deletion 5q)
Pomalidomide	Multiple myeloma

Abbreviation: FDA, U.S. Food and Drug Administration.

How do the IMiDs work?

- IMiDs work by directly inducing apoptosis, enhancing T-cell and natural killer (NK) cell–mediated cytotoxicity, inhibiting the production of proinflammatory cytokines (eg, interleukin 6 [IL-6], tumor necrosis factor alpha [TNF-alpha]), and inhibiting angiogenesis

- In multiple myeloma, the efficacy of the IMiDs is now thought to be related to the binding of these agents to cereblon, a protein of the E3 ubiquitin ligase complex. Binding of the IMiDs to cereblon leads to the enhancement of ubiquitination and degradation of transcription factors (Ikaros and Ailos) important in B-cell development

What are the common dosing ranges for the IMiDs?

- Thalidomide: 200 to 400 mg orally (PO) once daily

- Lenalidomide: 25 mg PO once daily days 1 to 21 of a 28-day cycle or days 1 to 14 of a 21-day cycle; 10 mg PO once daily for patients with myelodysplastic syndrome (MDS) with deletion 5q

- Pomalidomide: 4 mg PO once daily days 1 to 21 of a 28-day cycle

Are the IMiDs metabolized/eliminated renally or hepatically?

- Thalidomide: no dose adjustments necessary for hepatic or renal impairment

- Lenalidomide: eliminated renally—dose adjust for renal dysfunction

- Pomalidomide: metabolized in the liver—dose adjust for hepatic dysfunction

Are there drug interactions with any of the IMiDs?

- Pomalidomide: drugs that modulate the CYP3A4 and 1A2 pathway (the primary enzymes that metabolize pomalidomide; CYP2C19 and 2D6 also contribute to a lesser degree) may increase or decrease pomalidomide concentrations; drugs that inhibit or induce P-glycoprotein (P-gp) may increase or decrease pomalidomide concentrations, respectively.

What are the most common adverse effects of the IMiDs?

Most Common Adverse Effects of IMiDs

	Thalidomide	Lenalidomide	Pomalidomide
Myelosuppression	++	+++	+++
Embryo-fetal toxicity	+++	+++	+++
DVT/PE	+++	++	+
Neuropathy	+++	−	+
Constipation	+++	++	++

(continued)

Most Common Adverse Effects of IMiDs (*continued*)

	Thalidomide	Lenalidomide	Pomalidomide
Rash	+ +	+ +	+ +
Fatigue/sedation	+ + +	+	+ +

Notes: − does not typically occur, + rare, + + occasional, + + + common.

Abbreviations: DVT, deep vein thrombosis; ImiD, immunomodulatory agent; PE, pulmonary embolism.

What is the significance of the REMS programs associated with the IMiDs?

• There are risk evaluation and mitigation strategies (REMS) programs associated with each of the IMiDs—the goal is to prevent the risk of embryo-fetal exposure and to educate on the serious risks of these agents

• The prescriber, patient, and pharmacy must all be enrolled in the REMS programs and agree to comply with all requirements

• Full, specific requirements are available on the Celgene website

  – Thalidomide—www.thalomidrems.com

  – Lenalidomide—www.revlimidrems.com

  – Pomalidomide—www.pomalystrems.com

• Highlights of the program:

  – Prescribers enroll and certify for the REMS program

  – Prescribers counsel patients on benefits, risks, and appropriate contraception

  – Prescribers verify negative pregnancy test for females of reproductive potential

  – After completion of a patient-physician agreement form and mandatory prescriber/patient confidential survey, an authorization number is obtained for each prescription. This authorization number is written on the prescription, along with the patient risk category

  – Prescribers may write for no more than a 28-day supply at a time (no refills); prescriptions are sent to a certified pharmacy

– The pharmacy obtains a confirmation number from Celgene, counsels the patient, and completes an education and counseling checklist with the patient, prior to dispensing (along with a medication guide)

What is the emetogenicity level of the IMiDs?

• The IMiDs have minimal to low emetogenic risk

L-Asparaginase Enzymes

What are the chemotherapy agents in the asparaginase enzyme class?

- Pegaspargase (Oncaspar®)

- Asparaginase *Erwinia chrysanthemi* (Erwinaze®), also known as "Erwinia"

What malignancy are the asparaginase enzymes approved for?

- Acute lymphoblastic leukemia (ALL)

How do the asparaginase enzymes work?

- Lymphoblasts lack the enzyme asparagine synthetase and require exogenous asparagine for survival.

- Asparaginase cleaves asparagine into aspartic acid and ammonia, thus reducing the asparagine pool available for lymphoblast growth and protein synthesis, leading to apoptosis in these cells; asparaginase enzymes also have glutaminase activity, which may be responsible for their cytotoxicity as well.

- L-asparaginase products are derived from bacteria; pegaspargase is derived from *Escherichia coli* and Erwinia is derived from *Erwinia chrysanthemi*.

- Erwinia was developed for patients with hypersensitivity to *E. coli*–derived formulations; patients with allergic reactions or antibody formation toward the *E. coli*–derived products do not cross-react with Erwinia.

- Pegaspargase is a pegylated enzyme product and has a significantly longer half-life than Erwinia (5–12 days vs. ~16 hours);

pegylation of pegaspargase is also thought to reduce immunogenicity compared to the historical, non-pegylated, *E. coli*–derived asparaginase product (no longer on the market), potentially reducing allergic reactions and formation of antibodies to the product.

What are the common dosing ranges for the asparaginase enzymes?

- Pegaspargase: 1,000 to 2,500 units/m^2 intramuscular (IM) or intravenous (IV) (some protocols cap the dose at 1 vial or 3,750 units); do not administer more frequently than every 14 days

- Erwinia:

  – As a substitute for pegaspargase: 25,000 units/m^2 IM or IV three times weekly for six doses for each planned pegaspargase dose

  – As a substitute for asparaginase (*E. coli*): 25,000 units/m^2 IM or IV for each planned asparaginase (*E. coli*) dose

Are the asparaginase enzymes metabolized/eliminated renally or hepatically?

- The asparaginase enzymes are not eliminated hepatically or renally. Because of hepatotoxicity with asparaginase, caution is warranted in those with preexisting liver dysfunction.

Are there drug interactions with any of the asparaginase enzymes?

- Methotrexate—Asparaginase enzymes also display potent glutaminase activities. Methotrexate's activity depends on polyglutamation for optimal accumulation and activity within cancer cells. Thus, administration of asparaginase prior to methotrexate is antagonistic. In contrast, administration of methotrexate prior to asparaginase may be synergistic (eg, MOAD regimen for ALL).

What are the most common adverse effects of the asparaginase enzymes?

- Hypersensitivity reactions—urticaria, erythema, edema, chills, fever, rash, anaphylaxis

  – Can premedicate with diphenhydramine, acetaminophen, and corticosteroids

– Silent inactivation and antibody formation to asparaginase enzymes may occur even in the absence of clinical hypersensitivity

– In the case of anaphylaxis and/or severe hypersensitivity reactions, patients should be switched to an alternative asparaginase product (eg, switching pegaspargase [*E. coli* derived] to *Erwinia*-derived asparaginase)

- Hepatotoxicity
- Thrombosis and hemorrhage
- Hypertriglyceridemia
- Pancreatitis

- The "asparaginase blues"—fatigue, malaise, depression thought to be due to hyperammonemia

- Nausea/vomiting—more common with Erwinia given intravenously; this is thought to be due to rapid formation of high peak levels of ammonia

What is "silent inactivation" and why is this important with asparaginase enzymes?

- Silent inactivation refers to the development of autoantibodies to asparaginase products without evidence of clinical hypersensitivity; clinical hypersensitivity and development of autoantibodies do not correlate well.

- The development of autoantibodies may result in accelerated clearance of asparaginase, preventing asparagine depletion and efficacy of the product.

- In the case of silent inactivation to pegaspargase (*E. coli* derived), patients may be switched to *Erwinia*-derived asparaginase without cross-reactivity, allowing continued asparagine depletion in these patients, essential for optimal outcomes in ALL.

- To monitor for inactivation of asparaginase products, monitoring of asparaginase activity levels is necessary. The exact value is controversial; however, targeting nadir serum asparaginase activity levels of >0.2 international units/mL has been associated with optimal asparagine depletion.

What is the emetogenicity level of the asparaginase enzymes?

- Both agents are categorized as minimal (<10% frequency)

Are the asparaginase enzymes vesicants or irritants?

- Pegaspargase and Erwinia are neither vesicants nor irritants

16

Promyelocytic Leukemia Gene Retinoic Acid Receptor-Alpha (PML-RARα) Translocation Inhibitors

What are the agents in the PML-RARα inhibitor class?

• Tretinoin/all-trans retinoic acid (ATRA) (Vesanoid®) and arsenic tri-oxide (Trisenox®)

What malignancies are each PML-RARα inhibitor FDA approved for?

FDA-Approved Uses of PML-RARα Inhibitors

Agent	FDA Approval
ATRA	Acute promyelocytic leukemia (APL)
Arsenic trioxide	APL

Abbreviations: ATRA, all-trans retinoic acid; FDA, U.S. Food and Drug Administration.

How do the PML-RARα inhibitors work?

• The PML-RARα gene fusion results from a balanced translocation involving the PML gene on chromosome 15 and the RARα gene on chromosome 17. The product of this gene fusion binds with genetic promoters and recruits corepressor complexes, which repress normal gene expression and prevents differentiation of promyelocytes

• ATRA: causes the corepressor complexes to dissociate from RARα and allows for transcription and therefore differentiation of promyelocytes

- Arsenic trioxide: creates reactive oxygen species and degrades PML; creates intermolecular disulfide cross-links, which leads to multimerization and SUMOylation (a posttranslational modification) of PML; proteasome-dependent degradation occurs

What are the common dose ranges for each PML-RARα inhibitor?

- ATRA: 45 mg/m^2/day divided BID orally (with meals)
- Arsenic: 0.15 mg/kg/day intravenously

Are the PML-RARα inhibitors metabolized/eliminated renally or hepatically?

- Both agents are metabolized hepatically and renally eliminated

Are there drug interactions with any of the PML-RARα inhibitors?

- ATRA will have drug interactions with cytochrome P450 inhibitors/inducers (ATRA is also an inducer and induces its own metabolism)
- Arsenic: avoid QT prolonging agents

What are the major adverse effects of the PML-RARα inhibitors?

- ATRA: differentiation syndrome, hyperleukocytosis, headache, malaise, dizziness, hypercholesterolemia, hypertriglyceridemia, hepatotoxicity, skin rash, skin/mucous membrane dryness, pseudotumor cerebri, teratogenicity (boxed warning)
- Arsenic: differentiation syndrome, hyperleukocytosis, headache, QT prolongation (EKG twice weekly is recommended), potassium and magnesium wasting, skin rash, facial edema, peripheral neuropathy, musculoskeletal pain, hepatotoxicity, teratogenicity

What is differentiation syndrome?

- A relatively frequent complication of differentiating agent therapy (eg, arsenic trioxide, ATRA) in patients with APL, characterized by dyspnea, fever, weight gain, pulmonary infiltrates, pleural effusions, pericardial effusions, acute renal failure; may be fatal

- Treatment: Dexamethasone 10 mg BID; usually can continue ATRA and arsenic (in severe cases, both agents should be discontinued)

What is the emetogenicity level of the PML-RARα inhibitors?

- ATRA is categorized as minimal to low
- Arsenic is categorized as moderate emetic risk

Are the PML-RARα inhibitors vesicants or irritants?

- Arsenic is an irritant

III

Miscellaneous Oncolytics

17

Sipuleucel-T (Provenge®)

What malignancy is sipuleucel-T approved for?

- Metastatic castration-resistant prostate cancer

How does sipuleucel-T work?

- Sipuleucel-T is an autologous, dendritic cell–based immunotherapy directed against prostate cancer cells

- The patient undergoes leukopheresis to remove white blood cells, including antigen-presenting cells (APCs)

- The APCs are exposed to a fusion protein antigen consisting of prostatic acid phosphatase (PAP) (expressed on >95% of prostate cancers) linked to granulocyte-macrophage colony-stimulating factor (GM-CSF)

- Antigen is processed and presented on the surface of the APCs. GM-CSF acts to help stimulate APC activity

- The activated APC product is infused into the patient. Upon infusion, the activated APCs present the PAP antigen to T cells, leading to T-cell activation and proliferation toward prostate cancer cells expressing PAP

What is the dose of sipuleucel-T?

- ≥50 million CD54+ cells intravenously (IV) every 2 weeks × three doses

Is sipuleucel-T metabolized/eliminated renally or hepatically?

- Sipuleucel-T is neither eliminated renally nor metabolized hepatically

Are there drug interactions with sipuleucel-T?

- Concurrent immunosuppressive therapies may alter the efficacy of sipuleucel-T

What premedications are required for sipuleucel-T?

- Acetaminophen
- Diphenhydramine

What are the most common adverse effects of sipuleucel-T?

- Infusion-related reactions (usually within the first 24 hrs after administration)
  - Chills, fever, bronchospasm, hypertension, and so on
- Nausea, vomiting
- Myalgias and an influenza-like illness
- Headache, dizziness
- Citrate toxicity (due to the apheresis procedure)

What is the emetogenicity level of sipuleucel-T?

- Although not in the 2015 National Comprehensive Cancer Network (NCCN) antiemetic guidelines, sipuleucel-T would be categorized as low

Is sipuleucel-T a vesicant or irritant?

- Sipuleucel-T is neither a vesicant nor an irritant

18

Omacetaxine (Synribo®)

What malignancy is omacetaxine approved for?

- Chronic myeloid leukemia (CML), chronic or accelerated phase

How does omacetaxine work?

- Omacetaxine is an inhibitor of protein synthesis; thus, it does not require binding to the breakpoint cluster region-Abelson murine leukemia viral oncogene homolog 1 (BCR-ABL) kinase in CML and has activity against tyrosine kinase inhibitor–resistant BCR-ABL mutations (including the T315I mutation)

- Omacetaxine is a homoharringtonine derivative that binds to the A-site cleft on the ribosome, inhibiting protein synthesis by preventing amino acid chain elongation

- This action rapidly reduces short-lived proteins, including the BCR-ABL protein and others crucial for proliferation and cell survival (eg, C-myc, Mcl-1, Cyclin D1, XIAP)

What is the normal dose of omacetaxine?

- Induction: 1.25 mg/m^2 subcutaneously twice daily × 14 days (until achievement of hematologic response; every 28 days)

- Maintenance: 1.25 mg/m^2 subcutaneously twice daily × 7 days (every 28 days)

Is omacetaxine metabolized/eliminated renally or hepatically?

- Omacetaxine is not metabolized hepatically nor is the drug renally eliminated

Are there drug interactions with omacetaxine?

- No significant drug interactions have been characterized for omacetaxine

What are the most common adverse effects of omacetaxine?

- Myelosuppression
- Hyperglycemia
- Nausea/diarrhea (typically mild)
- Injection site reactions
- Arthralgia
- Fatigue

What is the emetogenicity level of omacetaxine?

- Omacetaxine has low emetogenic risk

19

Estramustine (Emcyt®)

What malignancy is estramustine approved for?

- Progressive or metastatic prostate cancer

How does estramustine work?

- Estramustine is a carbamate-linked conjugate of nor-nitrogen mustard (an alkylating agent) and estradiol

- It was synthesized on the premise that the estradiol component would bind to the estrogen receptor in breast cancer cells and selectively deliver the alkylating agent, nor-nitrogen mustard; however, it was neither found to have clinical activity in breast cancer, nor did it demonstrate alkylating agent activity

- Estramustine instead accumulates in the prostate by binding to a prostate-specific protein and inhibits microtubule function in prostate cancer cells

- Estramustine is cell cycle specific to the G2/M phase

What is the usual dose of estramustine?

- 14 mg/kg/day orally in 3 to 4 divided doses

Is estramustine metabolized/eliminated renally or hepatically?

- Estramustine is eliminated hepatically

Are there drug interactions with estramustine?

- Absorption of estramustine can be significantly decreased by coadministration with calcium (including antacids) and calcium-rich foods; patients should take estramustine on an empty stomach, at least 1 hour before or 2 hours after eating.

What are the most common adverse effects of estramustine?

- Nausea, vomiting, and diarrhea
- Gynecomastia, breast tenderness, decreased libido
- Fluid retention
- Increased liver enzymes
- Thromboembolism, congestive heart failure (CHF), myocardial infarction (MI) (rare, but serious)

What is the emetogenicity level of estramustine?

- Estramustine is categorized as moderate to high emetogenic risk

Appendix A: Agents Requiring Renal and/or Hepatic Dose Adjustments

Hepatic	Renal
All taxanes	NOT taxanes
All anthracyclines	NOT anthracyclines (except epirubicin)
All vinca alkaloids	NOT vinca alkaloids
NOT platinums	All platinums
All-trans retinoic acid (ATRA)	ATRA
Altretamine	Altretamine
Arsenic trioxide	Arsenic trioxide
5-Fluorouracil	Bleomycin
Belinostat	Capecitabine
Bendamustine	Carmustine
Bortezomib	Cladribine
Busulfan	Clofarabine
Carfilzomib	Cyclophosphamide
Carmustine	Cytarabine ($>200 \text{ mg/m}^2$)
Chlorambucil	Dacarbazine
Cyclophosphamide	Dactinomycin
Cytarabine	Etoposide
Dacarbazine	Fludarabine
Dactinomycin	Hydroxyurea

(*continued*)

(continued)

Hepatic	Renal
Estramustine	Ifosfamide
Etoposide	Lenalidomide
Ifosfamide	Lomustine
Irinotecan	Melphalan (only high doses)
Lomustine	Mercaptopurine
Mercaptopurine	Methotrexate
Methotrexate	Mitomycin
Mitomycin	Nelarabine
Panobinostat	Pemetrexed
Pomalidomide	Pentostatin
Procarbazine	Pralatrexate
Romidepsin	Streptozocin
Streptozocin	Temozolomide
Teniposide	Thiotepa
Thioguanine	Thioguanine
Thiotepa	Topotecan
Vorinostat	

Appendix B: Extravasation Risk of Chemotherapeutic Agents

Vesicants	Irritants
Dactinomycin*	Abraxane (paclitaxel albumin
Daunorubicin*‡	bound)*
Doxorubicin*‡	Ado-trastuzumab*
Epirubicin*‡	Arsenic trioxide*
Idarubicin*‡	Bendamustine*#
Liposomal vincristine†$	Busulfan*
Mechlorethamine*#	Cabazitaxel
Mitomycin*	Carboplatin*
Mitoxantrone*	Carmustine (BCNU)*^
Vinblastine†$	Cladribine*
Vincristine†$	Cisplatin*#
Vinorelbine†$	Dacarbazine*
	Docetaxel*
	Doxorubicin liposomal*
	Etoposide†$
	Fluorouracil
	Gemcitabine
	Ixabepilone
	Ifosfamide*^
	Irinotecan*
	Melphalan
	Oxaliplatin†#
	Paclitaxel*

(*continued*)

(*continued*)

Vesicants	Irritants
	Streptozocin
	Teniposide[†$]
	Topotecan[*]

Antidote and local care: [*]topical cooling, [†]topical heat, [‡]dexrazoxane, [#]sodium thiosulfate, [$]hyaluronidase, [^]topical dimethyl sulfoxide (DMSO).

Management of Extravasation

1. Stop infusion and intravenous (IV) fluids. Leave IV catheter in place. Do not flush the extravasated IV catheter

2. Disconnect IV tubing from IV catheter

3. Attach small syringe and attempt to aspirate as much fluid as possible (drug, fluid in tissue) to clear IV catheter of chemotherapy

4. Estimate amount of drug that was extravasated

5. If peripheral IV, remove IV catheter—avoid pressure to site of extravasation; mark area of induration or swelling

6. Administer appropriate antidote, if needed. Apply topical cooling or heat if indicated as well (see table in preceding text). Rest and elevate extremity

7. Consider plastic surgery expert consultation depending on severity and agent extravasated

Specific Extravasation Interventions

1. Dexrazoxane

a. Dose: 1,000 mg/m^2 (max 2,000 mg) IV daily days 1 to 2,500 mg/m^2 (max 1,000 mg) day 3

b. Administration:

   i. First dose should be given within 6 hours of extravasation

   ii. IV infusion over 1 hour into a functioning IV line that is not affected by the extravasation (ideally in the opposite arm)

iii. Avoid cooling procedures within 15 minutes of dexrazoxane administration

iv. Do NOT use topical dimethyl sulfoxide (DMSO) if using dexrazoxane

2. DMSO (topical)

a. Dose/administration:

i. 50% solution, 1 to 2 mL onto a sterile gauze pad and gently apply to the skin surface of extravasated site every 8 hours × 7 days

3. Hyaluronidase

a. Dose: 150 international units subcutaneously

b. Administration:

i. Administer subcutaneously with a small needle (eg, 25 gauge), distributing dose around the perimeter of the extravasation site in four or more equal injections, pointing the medication inward toward the center of the extravasated site

ii. Do not rub site; use new needle for each injection given

4. Sodium thiosulfate

a. Dose: 10% solution, 4 mL diluted with 6 mL sterile water; 2 mL of a solution for:

i. Each mg of mechlorethamine or bendamustine suspected of extravasating

ii. Each 100 mg of cisplatin suspected of extravasating

b. Administration:

i. Administer subcutaneously with a small needle (eg, 25 gauge), distributing dose around the perimeter of the extravasation site in four or more equal injections, pointing the medication inward toward the center of the extravasated site

ii. Do not rub site; use new needle for each injection given

iii. Avoid pressure to site; allow to air-dry—do not cover the site

iv. Do not use topical DMSO if using dexrazoxane

Index

Printed in the United States
By Bookmasters